HYDROPATHY,

ETC. ETC.

I.—Vincent Priessnitz.

"Discover what will destroy life, and you are a great man—what will prolong it and you are an impostor! Discover some invention in machinery that will make the rich more rich, and the poor more poor, and they will build you a statue! Discover some mystery in art, that will equalise disparities, and they will pull down their houses to stone you."—*Bulwer.*

Priessnitz was born at Gräfenberg, October, 4th 1800. His father became blind in his nineteenth year, and remained so until his death, which took place in 1838, a period of thirty-two years, during fourteen of which his son was his guide. His mother was killed by a bull in 1821.

Priessnitz's family have been in possession of the estate he now owns, consisting of about 180 acres of land, for upwards of 200 years, so that a mistake arose in calling him a peasant, instead of a farmer's son, or yeoman of Silesia. Two centuries ago (1645), when the country was invaded by the Swedes, a soldier, attempting to carry off a female of the family, was pursued and slain by one of Priessnitz's ancestors on the spot now called the Priessnitz-Quelle (or spring). A tablet placed over the spring, commemorates this event.

Priessnitz was born, in what is now called the "stone house," (opposite the large establishment) which he inherited with the land.

He began dabbling in the Water-cure, when only twelve or thirteen years old. Having sprained his wrist, he pumped upon it and applied a wet bandage, which produced an *Ausschlag*, or eruption; he not knowing whether it would be beneficial or otherwise. The question was, however, soon decided; for the *sprain* was cured. Finding the same plan, in other sprains, cuts, and bruises invariably succeed, he recommended its adoption to his neighbours.

He next applied the wet bandage to swollen joints and local pains, and was gradually led to its application in gout and rheumatism. Observing that the wet bandage remained cold from want of heat in the part affected, he covered it with a dry one to prevent evaporation, and confine the heat. The appearance of eruption in many cases before amelioration or cure, led him to suppose that there was generally some peccant or foreign matter required to be drawn out, or eliminated. Thus drawn on to think and reason on the subject, his powers of invention were kept in constant activity to find new expedients for producing the desired effects in the fresh cases presented to him; until the present complete and efficacious system, or science was gradually developed and matured.

In treating a cut hand in one person he found it heal kindly; in another, it became angry and inflamed: whence he concluded that the blood of the one was healthy, and of the other impure. Reflecting on the effect of bandages and baths, in extracting and attracting heat, and exciting eruptions when applied, he resorted to the elbow bath, and bandages up the arm, to relieve the hand. Other modes of treatment were progressively discovered and added.

When sixteen years of age, after loading a waggon with hay, Priessnitz was standing at the horse's head, whilst his companions were cogging the wheel; before this was effected the horse struggled, overcame him and rushed down the hill, which was very steep. Unwilling that the animal should destroy itself, Priessnitz would not relinquish his hold, his foot caught in a bush and he fell between the horse's feet, was dragged, trampled upon and severely bruised. He was taken up senseless, with two of his front teeth gone, and three ribs on the left side broken, he was carried home, and a doctor sent for: who, after causing great pain by probing and *punching* the side, applied his remedies, at the same time prognosticating that his patient would never perfectly recover. Priessnitz having no respect for treatment or opinion, declined the doctor's further attendance.

He then began to manage himself. By frequently holding his breath, and pressing his abdomen on the side of a table, for a painful length of time, he forced back the ribs into their proper position. Wet bandages were constantly applied and changed, and water drunk in abundance. By perseverance in these means he rapidly mended, and in twelvemonths his health was completely restored.

His own faith and that of many of his neighbours in the power of water was thus established; and ere long the peasantry from all sides flocked to him for aid. Some thought him endowed with the power of witchcraft; others honored him as a prophet; all wondering at his success in curing disease. Sponges used by him in washing his patients were regarded as talismans—as containing within them something gifted with a mysterious and marvellous operation. Broom-sticks were placed across his doorway, to see whether on coming out he could get over without displacing them, it being a prevalent opinion that only those practising witchcraft can.

His antagonists took advantage of this disposition of the people; and their opinion that Priessnitz was possessed by an evil spirit was encouraged by the priests, who denounced him publicly in the church. Some idea of the excitement got up against him may be found, from the fact, that the peasantry were in the habit of throwing stones at the early visitors to his house.

Numbers, however, came to him for advice, which he then only gave at his own house; afterwards he was induced to visit his patients. This seemed to dissolve the spell, and his reputation began to decline, notwithstanding he claimed no remuneration nor accepted any fee: from hundreds his applicants fell off to tens. He soon perceived that what is simple, costing neither money nor trouble, loses its value, or is but coldly appreciated; he therefore returned to his previous usage of giving advice only at home, leaving people to believe as much as they pleased in the magical virtues of his remedies.

His reputation now rose higher than ever, and spread far and wide. Strangers from distant parts came to Gräfenberg, so that he was compelled to increase the size of his house for their accommodation; and thus his establishment commenced.

He was not yet, however, allowed to proceed smoothly in his career: many viewed his growing reputation with jealousy. The two medical men and the Burgomaster at Freiwaldau set on foot a conspiracy to crush him. Their persecutions lasted thirteen years: but, as frequently occurs in similar cases, these were among the circumstances that eventually advanced his success; since but for this pressure from without, he never would have so completely developed the power of water over disease; and the physiological and pathological truths that have in consequence come to light, must still have lain buried in darkness. During all this period, he was strictly watched, to see if he applied aught else than the pure element; calling for the exertion of his utmost ingenuity, to supply, by water alone, the place of every other remedy.

He was frequently brought before the Syndic at Freiwaldau; but all endeavours to convict him of any unlawful act (which the administration of drugs or herbs in an unlicensed practitioner would have been) had failed, when in 1828, a more determined attempt was made to put an end to his proceedings. Witnesses were brought forward to prove that he had injured them, and others that he had pretended to cures that had actually been performed by the medical men. But none, when examined, could deny that Priessnitz had benefited them, and taken no payment in return.

There was a miller, whom both the doctor and Priessnitz claimed the merit of curing. On being examined, the miller was asked which of the two had effected the cure? "What shall I say?" answered he: "*Both*; the doctor relieved me of my money, and Priessnitz of my disease. In return, I have given him nothing—not even thanks, which I take this opportunity of offering him for the first time." This was of little avail; his calumniators had resolved his downfall. Accordingly, he was next accused of quackery, in illegally tampering with the public health, and ordered to be put under arrest. An appeal to the tribunal at Brünn, caused this unjust sentence to be reversed; and he then obtained permission to have a cold-water bathing establishment. Discontented at this, his persecutors shortly after brought him to the court at Weidenau, a neighbouring town, on the hypocritical plea that the connection between his accusers and the authorities of Freiwaldau might, contrary to their wishes, give a colour of unfairness to the proceedings. The tribunal of Weidenau could not reverse the sentence of that at Brünn, but prohibited Priessnitz from treating any persons but those of his own parish or district. He replied that water was free to all, and that he was not in the habit of inquiring whence an invalid came previously to administering aid. Feeling he was right, he persisted in acting as before; and for some time, no further notice was taken of him.

In 1831, his enemies took a bolder course, by raising an alarm of the craft being in danger. This enlisted in their cause the medical men at Vienna, who brought the subject under the notice of the emperor. He sent Dr. Baron Turckheim with a commission of district and staff surgeons to Gräfenberg, to investigate and report on the new system, and the proceedings of its originator. Notwithstanding that most of these gentlemen were prejudiced against both, they were astonished and pleased at what they witnessed; and their report was of so favourable a nature, that Priessnitz was allowed by imperial authority to carry on his establishment, with the addition of the privilege enjoyed by staff surgeons of giving sick certificates to public employés and officers under his care. This state of things was, however, again shortly afterwards disturbed. In 1835, the emperor Francis being dead, fresh intrigues induced the government authorities at Troppau (a town about fifty miles from Gräfenberg) to withdraw the permission Priessnitz had received for giving sick certificates. He was urged to appeal to the higher powers, but declined, saying—"The matter must right itself," and steadily refused giving sick certificates, even to foreign officers. These complained, through their ambassadors, to the authorities at Vienna; and for them, Priessnitz's power of granting certificates was restored. The Austrian officers and employés being still excluded, also exerted themselves through friends in the capital; and the matter was, in the end, satisfactorily arranged.

In 1843, the Prussian government, doubtless under medical influence, forbade all officers or employés proceeding to any hydropathic establishment out of Prussia, unless expressly recommended by their medical advisers.

The greatest difficulty in obtaining passports to the Hygiean temple is also encountered by the Russian Poles. It has been observed by many from both these countries who, nevertheless, reached Gräfenberg, that their medical men strongly recommended their not going to Priessnitz, and willingly gave certificates for any other establishment, even though in a foreign country.

For thirty years, although all publications against Priessnitz and the Water-cure were tolerated in the Austrian dominions, none in favour of either were permitted. But, as though willing to do tardy justice and urged on by public opinion, in July, 1845, the Vienna Gazette inserted a favourable article on both subjects.

From the age of seven to twenty-one, Priessnitz was in constant attendance on his blind father; and on that account, escaped the liability of being drawn as a soldier. Early in life he married a distant relation of his own name, daughter of the *Schulz* or chief magistrate of Bömishdorf, who was by trade a miller. He has had nine children, of whom six daughters and one son are living. The first-born, a sickly boy, died of apoplexy. When taken ill, the wife and relations insisted on having a physician from Nicholasdorf: this was at the commencement of Priessnitz's career, and he reluctantly yielded. He has since said he would not have given way, had he imagined the doctor could have killed the child so soon, for a powerful medicine being administered, death was the almost immediate result. Priessnitz supposes it was calomel. Whatever it was, it produced spasms and death.

This was a severe lesson to Mrs. Priessnitz, who since that event has left the treatment of her children entirely to her husband.

As has been said, the various manipulations which now form so complete a system, were gradually introduced just as Priessnitz became aware of their necessity and had experience of their effect.

Finding that pain was relieved by natural perspiration, he instituted the sweating process by covering the patients up well in bed. Some time later he improved on this, by introducing the blankets. On a patient becoming faint, whilst under the process, he found that opening the windows to admit fresh air, and washing the face, afforded relief, and ordered it with equal advantage generally. At first he sponged the throat, then the chest, and gradually the whole body; finding the extension of this practice most beneficial in *every* case, he ventured on the tepid (*i. e.* 62° Fahr.) bath and ultimately the plunge or cold bath.

The relief afforded by local bandages to the finger, arm, leg, and other parts of the body afflicted with pain, or to which he wished to attract the vicious juices, suggested the use of the waist bandage, which he found fulfilled many useful purposes, especially in relieving pain in the abdomen, feverishness, and restlessness, and also in bringing the abdominal functions into a healthy state.

Satisfied of the benefit derived from local cold bandages, he thought they might be extended over the whole of the surface of the body; and this originated the wet sheet, which supersedes the lancet by relieving the overcharged system of heat, and is the most powerful sedative known. It has gradually superseded the sweating process, though not in all cases. Priessnitz recommended the weaker patients to remain in the blanket only a sufficient time to get thoroughly warm; but they, thinking to accelerate a cure, sometimes remained in it too long, and fainted from exhaustion—a reason assigned for confining his treatment more especially to the wet sheet.

In chronic cases, which resisted the application of bandages, tepid and cold baths, he long tried local baths, to cause internal excitement and reaction; thence arose the hip, arm, foot, and head baths, which were generally successful: but in some obstinate cases, where they were not so, Priessnitz wished for a more powerful agent, and hit upon the douche, to which his attention was drawn by reflecting on the benefit he had received by pumping on his sprained wrist.

The rubbing sheet is a much later addition, being an improvement on rubbing with wet hands, or using sponges. It is a means of rousing latent heat, and administering an ablution to delicate persons, who could not endure an immersion in the bath.

This combination of novel and invaluable appliances will effect any purpose attempted by the pharmacopœia. In fact, so complete and efficacious is the system, that it may justly be termed a science putting into the shade all hygeian discoveries from the days of Hippocrates to the present time.

"Notwithstanding there are several defects in point of beauty, and a sternness of outline in almost every feature," there is something in the whole expression of Priessnitz's countenance peculiarly pleasing as well as striking; and one reads there kindness of heart as well as firmness and decision.

Among all his neighbours, his character stands deservedly high. From his infancy, he has been a pattern of sobriety and virtue, a good Christian, kind neighbour, an excellent husband and father; ever prompt to acts of benevolence and, though secretly, to acts of charity. Poverty deprives no invalid of his succour. Many, for months together, enjoy the hospitality of his table, and benefit by his advice, who have no means of making any pecuniary return. Indeed, Priessnitz never demands a fee, nor complains if none be given. Nevertheless, he has become rich by the exercise of prudence and economy.

It is worthy of record, that he never wrote a line or caused anything to be inserted in newspapers on the subject of his discoveries, or employed any of the means of publicity usually resorted to make known his establishment; yet this is frequented by denizens of all nations, and his fame extends to the antipodes.

When the author went to Gräfenberg in 1841, there seemed a deficiency of English; of whom he found but three. There were members of every grade of society from the crowned head to the beggar, all submitting themselves to Priessnitz's directions.

Anxious to make my countrymen acquainted with a system which had benefited thousands, and from which I had personally derived great advantage, immediately on my return home I published a work suggested by my visit to Gräfenberg, which proved to be actually the first that had appeared in England on the subject. Many English were thus induced to undertake a journey to see Priessnitz, and several books shortly afterwards came out, attesting the writer's high opinion of his skill, with their faith in the efficacy of his method. The number of English pilgrims to the Hygeian temple increased; and it is at present one of their favorite resorts. In 1848, a letter numerously signed was sent to America, and was inserted in the *New York Tribune*.

"TO THE EDITOR OF THE TRIBUNE.

"SIR, *Gräfenberg, 14th August, 1849.*

"The undersigned, desirous to alleviate suffering, and to promote the health and comfort of human beings, wish to call attention to the Water-cure as practised by Vincent Priessnitz. Not a particle of medicine is ever administered in any form or quantity. No bleeding, blistering, or leeching is ever employed.

"It is not pretended that the Water-cure is a universal specific for all diseases; but there are sufficient facts to prove that all diseases curable, and many incurable by any known means, can be healed by a proper application of the Water-cure, which the following cases will demonstrate.

"Count Mitrowski, an Austrian nobleman, aged fifty-four, who had long been afflicted with gout, and whose name we are permitted to use, was found insensible in his bed in an apoplectic fit. Some medical men were quickly in attendance and Priessnitz was sent for. The professional men considered the Count past recovery; and one of them said that he would throw his drugs away and become an hydropathist if this patient was restored. It was proposed by some to bleed the invalid, to which Priessnitz objected, if he was to bear any part of the responsibility. So far gone was the patient, and so nearly extinct did vitality appear, that a priest administered the extreme unction, and according to the custom of the country, a lighted candle was placed in each hand of the apparently dead man. By cold water treatment alone under the sagacious direction of Priessnitz, this gentleman recovered consciousness on the *third day*, drove out in a phaeton on the fourth, and gradually returned to his former habits.

"The only son of a Sovereign Prince, aged three years, suffered for fifteen months from chronic obstruction of the bowels, which baffled the skill of his medical attendants, and resulted in total atrophy. For twenty-seven days the child had *had no relief*, when, by the physician's advice, Priessnitz was called in. He saw the child; and at his suggestion the Prince and his family came here, in order that Priessnitz might daily superintend the treatment. In a few days the disease yielded to the water-cure, and at the end of three months, the child returned quite well.

"A lady of rank suffered severely from frequent head-aches, cramp in the stomach, indigestion, and other maladies, which cannot here be particularised. She constantly threw up her food, even whilst in the act of eating, and could not have the slightest relief without medicine, and even then had great pain and difficulty. She had been under medical treatment for fourteen years, during which time she consulted fourteen eminent physicians. In little more than a year under the Water-cure, she was restored to perfect health.

"A gentleman had one of the worst attacks of small-pox, complicated with measles. From the fact of his vomiting blood any medical man will judge of the malignity of the disease.

"In a fortnight he was out of doors; and in four weeks all traces of the disease were rapidly disappearing.

"Here is one case of a gentleman advanced in life and long an invalid,—another of a tender infant,—a third of a lady,—a fourth of a person labouring under what is generally considered a fatal disease, and *all restored*.

"The undersigned trust you will kindly insert this statement, which they are impelled to offer from a desire to make known to others the benefit derivable from a system in the efficacy of which, as well as in the sagacity and skill of its founder Priessnitz they have the fullest confidence, and to which, humanly speaking, some of them owe their lives, and are,

"Sir,

"Your most obedient servants,

E. H. Tracey, the Hon., *England*
J. Hailes, Major, Bengal Army
Hugh Barr, *Paisley, Scotland*
J. H. O. Moore, Capt. H. B. M. S.

Edward Birch, British Consul

J. F. Sparkes, *England*
C. A. Lane, Lieut. Col., Bengal Army
Alonzo Draper, *New York*
T. V. Ganahl, *Inspruck, Tyrol*
C. W. Ganahl, *Ditto*
H. C. Wright, *Philadelphia, N. Y.*
H. D. Avrainville, *Ditto*
Baron Rudolph, *Lüttechan, Austria*
Count Guillaume D'Aichott, *Westphalia*
Charles Dr. Pickler, *Gratz, Styria*
Baron de Leutch, Capt. Austrian Army
Count Pierre, Dr., *Goess, Styria*
Baron Keller, Capt. Austrian Army
Count Zelenski, Chamberlain, *Austria*
Gustav Hirschfeld, *Holstein*
H. K. Marcher, M. D. *Denmark*
Count Wallowitz, *Poland*
L. Lemoile, French Consul
Baron de Wrede, *Austria*
Count Henkel, Dannesmark, *Prussia*
C. Balsch, Grand Logothet, *Moldavia*
Baron de Pabst, *Holland*
J. N. Spencer, Surgeon Dentist, *London*
F. B. Y. Ribas, Spanish Consul, *Odessa*
F. Harnish, Apothecary, *Bresslau*
Donilzi de Galetti, Capt., Russian Army
Alexr. de Harmasaki, *Moldavia*
V. Hake, Lieut. Col., *Prussia*
V. Crety, Lieut., *Ditto*
Otto Schramm, Royal Councillor, *Prussia*
Edward Hoffman, Lieut. Prussian S.
Edward Calvos. Lieut. Austrian S.
J. Gibbs, *Enniscorthy, Ireland*
Edward Joseph Tabelar, Councillor, *Vienna*
Baron C. V. Radzig, *Bavaria*
Michael Avrial, Merchant, *Paris*
Ignace St. de Ionnewald, Major, *Austria*
V. Siegl, Barrister, *Austria*

L. J. E. Rudnick, Phil. Doc., *Prussia*
E. C. Ellery, *London*
G. Pietsch, *Leeds*
Sig. Goetzel, *Vienna*
Count J. Schaffgotsch, Chamberlain to King of Prussia
Baron F. D'Unsulz, *Poland*
Baron Schmidburg, Sect. Austrian Gov.
A. B. Mills, *Glasgow*
J. T. Delvarnes, son of Ex-President of Chili
H. A. Muller, *Hambro'*
Carl Burmester, *Ditto*
H. Schierholz, *Ditto*
Theod. Heyman, *Ditto*
E. Holzmann, *Ditto*
Count Szirmay, Chamberlain, A. G.
H. G. Robinson, *Yorkshire*
L. de Grotoski, *Poland*
Napoleon Maleski, *Ditto*
J. Slatter, *Isle of Jersey*
Le Chevalier de Montiglio, Sec. Legation, *Sardinia*
Prince Auguste Ruspoli, *Rome*
F. Kronwald, Councillor, *Austria*
Count Zeno Sarav, Austrian Chamberlain
Baron Tindal, Sec. Legation, *Holland*
The Rev. Thos. Smythe, *England*
J. Hamilton, *Carnacassa, Monaghan, Ireland*
L. Bardel, Lieut. Austrian S.
H. de Strager, Lieut., *Ditto*
C. Niemann, Provincial Deputy, *Pomerania, Prussia*
Victor Kurnatowksi, *Poland*
Baron N. de Höpken, *Stockholm*
Genges Siebil, *Lyons, France*
Karl Quovos, *Prussian Poland*
Francis Rieger, *Cracow*
Johann Gotthilf, President Criminal Court, *Prussia*
Count Oscar Roswadowski, *Austria*
Baron J. Wallish, *Ditto*
Baron M. Lyncker, Lieut., *Prussia*

Baron Mezenthin, Major, *Ditto*

Ivan A. Roiz, *Brazils, S. America*
Nicholas Arnault, *Paris*
Guiseppe Weyher, *Trieste*
August Navez, Lieut., *Belgium*

V. de Lauken, Lieut. Prussian S.	Wilhelm Lommatsch, *Saxony*
V. Siegler, Capt. Austrian S.	Baron A. Ledderer, Colonel, *Austria*
Count V. Orosz, Sec. Excise Bureau, *Vienna*	Von Kutzl, Lieut., *Ditto*
V. Perboe, Lieut. Austrian S.	Von Bovelmo, Lieut., *Ditto*
L. Liebshang, Postmaster, *Austria*	Baron Huelberg, Lieut., *Ditto*

"P.S.—We, the undersigned, cannot vouch for the exactitude of each particular in the four cases, related above, not having been at Gräfenberg during their occurrence; but we are happy to state our conviction and experience to be fully in favor of this mode of treatment.

E. Hallman, M. D., *Berlin*	R. L. Jones, *Luton, Bedfordshire*
Peter Wilson, Writer to the Signet, *Scotland*	A. J. Colvin, *Albany, N. Y.*
Horatio Greenhough, *U. S.*	A. F. Webster, R. N., *Battle Abbey, Sussex*
A. Schrotterick, M. D., *Norway*	W. Cybulvo, M. D., *Prague*
Francisco Bazan, *de la Province de Seville en Espana*, M. D.	Dr. Hempin, *Prussia*
J. M. Gutterieg Estrada, late Plenipotentiary to the Court of London, from *Mexico*	W. Murray, *Monaghan, Ireland*
C. M. Mecker, *America*	W. S. Ellis, *Middle Temple, London*
	T. H. Cohen, *London*"

In 1845 a work of a very different tendency appeared, which, though approving of the hydropathic treatment in itself, denounced Priessnitz's application of it, and calumniated him personally in the most unwarrantable and groundless manner. The author was R. H. Graham, M. D.; and so unpardonable was his attack on Priessnitz that it drew forth the following letter.

"To the Editor of the London Times,

"Gräfenberg, 2nd February, 1845.

"Sir.—We, the undersigned British and Americans, who have resided here for periods varying from three months to two years and upwards, and who consequently have had ample opportunities of acquiring correct information, deem it our duty publicly to assert that a work, entitled 'A true Report of the Water-cure, by Robert Hay Graham, M.D.' abounds in gross exaggerations, mis-statements, and calumnies respecting Priessnitz. It would lengthen this document too much to go into a detailed repetition of all those portions of Dr. Graham's work which we could contradict; we therefore refrain from noticing any in particular: it will be sufficient to say, that *from personal observations,* we can deny several of Dr. Graham's allegations, and, from information upon which we *can* rely, we are convinced that many more are totally devoid of foundation.

"We have seen a letter dated January 15th, 1845, from Captain Wollf, whom Dr. Graham gives as his authority for some of his most unfounded assertions, and to whom he dedicates his book; and we beg attention to the following extracts from that letter.

"'I not only' says Captain Wolff, 'was a passionate Hydropathist, but am still, to this day, known as an out-and-out one ... the information which I gave Dr. Graham, concerned solely the scientific part of the Water-cure, and could not, of course, be otherwise than favourable; I being, as above stated, an Hydropathist. With regard to the wretched stuff you allude to, as to whether Mr. and Mrs. P. drink wine or grog, whether Miss J. S. and other English ladies were treated with or without clothes, the tiresome story about Munde, or whether the Princess L. did or did not employ the Water-cure, with such like, I have never concerned myself; for I lived at Gräfenberg exclusively for the Water-cure.'

"Thus does Dr. Graham's principal witness fail him! It is only necessary to add, that we do not place the least reliance on any of Dr. Graham's statements. We are led to say thus much from regard to truth, and from esteem for a great and good man, who has been basely vilified.

"In our opinion Priessnitz, from long practice, varied experience, and close observation, guided by his extraordinary genius, has acquired so intimate a knowledge of the action of water, of its dangers and advantages as regards the human body, both in health and disease, that the most delicate invalid may safely rely on his judgment; and in this opinion we are sustained by the fact of his great success in the treatment of almost every variety of disease, which surpasses that of any physicians on record. The patients who seek his aid may be divided, with few exceptions, into two classes:—those who by medical men have been pronounced incurable; and those, whose diseases are the result of medical treatment: and, out of the large number whom he yearly treats, it would be absurd to expect that he should never lose one.

But we cannot believe that the Water-cure is the best remedy for disease, without also believing that he, its discoverer, is the best practitioner of it; and to convince us to the contrary would require somewhat stronger and more unexceptionable testimony than that of Dr. Graham. From the portrait which Dr. Graham draws of Priessnitz, one who did not know him, would be apt to imagine him as full of assumption and Charlatanism, whereas he is as far from either as any man; being as remarkable for his simplicity and truth, as for a native modesty and unassuming propriety of demeanour, which, combined with his kindliness of heart, win respect and regard from almost all who approach him. Requesting that you will do us the favour to give insertion to this letter, We are, Sir, Your obedient Servants,

Lichfield (The Earl of)	Horatio Greenough, *U.S.*
E. H. Tracey (The Hon.)	W. D'Arley
W. S. Ellis, *Temple*	John Gibbs
Richard L. Jones	William Murray
Gretton Bright	Andrew J. Colvin, *U.S.*
Augustus Blair (Capt.)	Alonzo Draper, *U.S.*
J. H. O. Moore (Capt.)	G. Pietsch
Thomas Smithell, M.A.	James Hamilton
Andrew B. Mills	Henry J. Robinson
C. Sewell	C. H. Meeker, *U.S.*"

If Dr. Graham's object was to injure Priessnitz, it was, unquestionably thoroughly defeated; for his fame continued to increase, and at the end of the same year, Gräfenberg was honoured by a visit from the Archduke Charles, heir apparent to the imperial crown of Austria, who treated Priessnitz with the greatest consideration, and shewed great interest in the Hydropathic treatment. On his arrival, an address was presented to him, numerously signed by the visitors at Gräfenberg, and presented by—

Don I. M. Estrada, Ex-Minister from Mexico to London	Baron A. D. Lotzbeck, Chamberlain to the King of Bavaria
Count Cyacki, Grand Marshal of Poland.	Capt. Moore, 35th Regt.
Count Shaffgatch, Chamberlain to the King of Prussia	F. La. Moile, Ex-Consul de France.

The Archduke seemed much pleased with it; and as it was a novelty in Germany, where addresses are unknown, we think a translation may be interesting to our readers.

> *Address presented to* Archduke Franz Carl, *at Gräfenberg, October 4th, 1845.*

"We, the undersigned natives of various countries, enjoying here the hospitality and protection of a paternal government, hasten to take advantage of the propitious occasion offered by the presence of your Imperial and Royal Highness, to lay our homage at your feet. How could we fail to evince the sentiments of gratitude which we entertain towards your illustrious house, for the favour it has deigned to grant for the development of a system, which has produced such happy results on ourselves, on that around us, and on the thousands of invalids who have preceded us. The protection of Government having been extended to the establishment at Gräfenberg and Freiwaldau, your Royal and Imperial Highness has judged it not unworthy to see with your own eyes the marvellous effects of a treatment, which gradually spreading over the universe, will preserve the human race from the double curse of intemperance and disease. For this condescension we tender our thanks. In all times and in all countries the use of cold water as a curative means has been acknowledged. The great physicians of past ages already had recourse to it. Travellers relate singular cures effected by its means amongst even the most savage tribes. In recent times we occasionally see light feebly penetrating through the darkness of prejudice and routine, and revealing the neglected virtues of this simple gift of nature; but these facts remaining isolated, the germs of such a noble discovery had hitherto always remained undeveloped. It was reserved to the soil of Austria to give birth to the immortal author of a system which can already rank among the sciences. Priessnitz, a simple farmer, in a poor and retired hamlet, obeying only the promptings of his genius, has triumphed over all obstacles, and, still young, has marched with a rapid step towards the destiny of great men. Relying solely on observation and experience, he realised truths which the science of ages could not reveal. The fame of his marvellous cures resounded at first in the immediate neighbourhood: but his star always rising and never vacillating, at last ended by shining throughout the world. Invalids from the most remote countries hastened in great numbers to submit themselves implicitly to his directions. Many disciples of medicine even hesitated not to throw aside their prejudice, and become enlightened by his discoveries. His cottage became the refuge of suffering humanity, his hamlet the seat of a new doctrine; still, far from being intoxicated with so much success and such unexpected good fortune, Priessnitz has in no way deviated from his original simplicity and primitive manners. His greatest ambition is the accomplishment of the laborious task he has imposed on himself; his sweetest recompence the affection and veneration of all who surround him. We know not which to admire most, the rare genius of this gifted man, or the firmness and modesty which characterise him. Guided by gratitude, and the admiration we feel for the Hydropathic system and its origination, we have ventured to present this humble address to your Imperial and Royal Highness, trusting that the visit of such an enlightened Prince will be a good augury for the further dev[e]lopment and extension of the curative system from which we have ourselves experienced such happy results."

In the ensuing summer a most flattering testimony was decreed to Priessnitz by the Emperor of Austria. It was a gold medal (called a *Verdienst Medaille* or medal of merit), and was presented to him by the Governor of Troppau, on the 7th of July, 1846, at the altar, with great ceremony, in the very church in which he had been formerly denounced. Shortly after, an incident occurred which had nearly deprived the world of this great man: this was the marriage of his eldest daughter, then only seventeen, to an Hungarian nobleman of large fortune. The young couple started for Hungary; and Priessnitz, on taking leave of them, was observed to be much affected. Later in the day, whilst visiting his patients, he found it difficult to lift one hand to his head. He hurried home, where he hardly arrived when he was suddenly struck with general paralysis, and was quite insensible. His attendants resorted to his own remedies, he was placed in a tepid bath and rubbed by four persons for nearly two hours before he began to regain his senses, when he ordered the tepid water to be changed for cold; and he has since been heard to say, the former would not have been attended with sufficient reaction, and consequently would not have had the desired effect. He now ordered his own treatment and recovered in a few days; his health was afterwards re-established by a fortnight's visit to his daughter in Hungary.

A few months since he was rejoiced by the birth of a son. This event conferred great happiness on him; for, as may be remembered, his first-born whom he lost was a son, and all his other children until the last, were daughters.

It is to be hoped, that Providence will spare his valuable life to see his son grow up, so that he may initiate him experimentally in the theory of Hydropathy, which can never be perfectly disseminated in any other way.

Several monuments and fountains erected at Gräfenberg, testify the admiration and respect in which Priessnitz is held. The English and the Hamburghers are at present engaged in erecting similar testimonies. The latter have placed his bust in the Exchange at Hamburg.

Judging from the strides Hydropathy is making, it is fair to conclude that in the course of time these examples will be followed by every nation in the world.[1]

II.—Hydropathy.

The term "hydropathy," has been cavilled at; its etymological sense meaning "water-disease," whilst its conventional sense means "water-cure." If disposed to dispute about terms, we might say that "physiology," in its etymological sense, means merely a discourse about nature; whilst, in a conventional sense, we understand it to treat of the science of animal life. For want of a better word, that of "hydropathy" was adopted, to express the manner of curing disease, by cold and tepid general and local baths, wet sheets (sometimes called linen baths), dripping-sheets, douche and friction, air, exercise, and drinking water. To this may be added, simplicity in our habits, and temperance in our manner of living.

In fact, by the term "hydropathy," were intended all those appliances by which nature may be put in the best possible way of assisting herself, since no allopathist, homæopathist, or hydropathist, will pretend that anything he can administer has of itself any healing virtue. It is a common observation, that riding, climbing, and exercise, give us strength; the horses, hedges, mountains and ground, do not, however, impart strength, but they afford the opportunity, the necessary resistance to develop or increase that strength which is in us. The weak man, do what you will, can only develop the strength which is in him, and the strong man the same. Let, therefore, the reader judge which is best calculated to cause that development—hydropathy or drugs.

III.—What Does Hydropathic Treatment Effect?

It promotes the vital energies, quickens the action of the absorbents, strengthens the nerves, allays irritation, promotes healthy action of the vital organs.

The extreme vessels deposit healthy particles, which the absorbents remove.

Dr. Gibbs, in his "Letters from Gräfenberg," states that water, applied hydropathically, acts in the following ways:—

1st. By the more rapid liberation of caloric.

2nd. By accelerating the change of tissues.

3rd. By constringing the capillaries.

4th. By increasing nervous power.

5th. By restoring tone to the skin.

6th. By derivation.

7th. By forwarding the elimination of morbific matter; or, in other words, as a sedative, alterative, tonic, stimulant, derivative, and counter-irritant.

And taken internally, it acts—

1st. As a solvent, and contributes to the greater part of the transformations.

2nd. Gives tone to the stomach.

3rd. Promotes the secretions and excretions, particularly from the skin, bowels, and kidneys.

4th. It is a most important and indispensable element in the blood; and "its partial application," says Dr. Johnson, "acts by determining the force of oxygen from one part to another; it produces all the effects of bleeding and blistering—except the pain," and he might have added, the debility.

The hydropathic treatment causes the elimination of all foreign matters from the body, and thereby promotes contraction, without which there can be no health, which Dr. Billing has shewn to demonstration; he states "that the proximate cause of *all* disease is relaxation and enlargement of the capillaries: the indication of a cure, therefore, is to constringe the capillaries, and cause them to contract, and resume their healthy state."

"As all organic action is contraction, all organic or animal strength depends upon the power of the different parts of the body to contract." If it be true, that the effect to be brought about in the treatment of *all* disease is to unload and constringe the capillaries, how can this be better achieved than by the sweating or wet-sheet process, and the cold bath; Dr. Johnson says—"The hydropathic treatment, which unloads the capillaries by sweating, and constringes them by cold, is clearly an efficient substitute for bleeding, purging, vomiting, uva ursi, digitalis, antimony, mercury, arsenic, nitrate of silver, sulphate of copper, iodine, iron, and multitudes of other remedies, enumerated by Dr. Billing, merely by their power of unloading and constringing the capillaries."

Priessnitz's theory:—

1st. That by the hydropathic treatment, the bad juices are brought to, and discharged by, the skin.

2nd. A new circulation is given to the diseased or inactive organs, and better juices infused into them.

3rd. All the functions of the body are brought into a normal state, not by operating upon any particular function, but upon the whole.

If these are the results of hydropathy—and that they are so, has never been disputed; nay, the truth is even proved by the following great medical authority unconnected with the water cure: it must be admitted that the sooner drugs are dispensed with the better.

British and Foreign Medical Review, and Quarterly Journal, October, 1846.—Extract.

"The water cure is a *stomachic*, since it invariably increases the appetite.

"It is a *local calefacient* in the wet sheet covered by a dry one.

"It is a *derivative*; cold friction at one part, by *exciting increased action there, producing corresponding diminution elsewhere; the compress* frequently acting, if not like a blister, at least *like a mustard poultice.*

"*It is a local as well as a general counter-irritant.*

"*It is essentially alterative* in the continual removal of old matter: its renewal is shewn in the maintenance of the same weight.

"An important hydropathic principle is, that almost all its *measures are applied to the surface.* One of the most formidable difficulties with which the ordinary physician has to contend is, that nearly all his remedies reach the point to which they are directed *through one channel.*

"The only means of relieving certain diseases is *by inundating the stomach* and bowels with foreign and *frequently* to them *pernicious substances.*

"Hydropathy employs a system of most extensive energetic general and local counter irritation.

"A fifth physiological feature of hydropathy is the number of coolings. The *generation of caloric has been traced to its right source*. It results from the burning up of waste matter, which by accumulation would become injurious.

"It is singular enough that almost all arguments used against cold bathing are the strongest theoretical arguments in its favor. Dr. Baynard, a most sarcastic writer, gives us the following anecdote:—

"Here a demi-brained doctor of more note than *nous,* asked, in the amazed agony of his half-understanding, how 'twas possible that an external application should affect the bowels, and cure pain within? 'Why doctor,' quoth an old woman standing by, 'by the same reason that, being wet-shod or catching cold from without, should give you the gripes and pain within.'

"If a rude exposure of the surface to cold and wet is capable of producing internal disease, there is no *doubt that a close relation exists between these agents and the morbid* conditions of internal parts."

After devoting upwards of thirty pages to prove the value of Hydropathy, the reviewer sums up as follows:—

"After what has been said and written in favor of Hydropathy.—*Judgment must therefore be entered by default against its opponents, and hydropathy is entitled to the verdict of harmlessness, since cause has never been shown to the contrary.*"

IV.—How are the Effects described in the last Chapter produced?

Are the effects, as described by hydropathists and by the British and Foreign Medical Review, produced without purging, vomiting, drugging, or the lancet—or by what other means are such essential results to be attained? We answer, by hydropathy alone are they to be produced, through the medium of the external and internal skin or mucous membrane, the most important organ in the human structure, and the most neglected by the guardians of the public health; and by the promotion of all the secretions and excretions.

The Abbé Sanctorius, a Florentine, might be said to have spent twenty years of his life in a balance determining the amount of matters thrown off by the pores of the skin. To ascertain this, he first cleaned and then placed small glasses, some not longer than thimbles, on various parts of the human frame, when the result proved that every man ought to pass off from his person, daily, from six to seven pounds. Two and a half pounds are supposed to be released by the ordinary modes of evacuation, and the remainder by the pores of the skin. Now, if this exhalation is impeded, and the necessary amount not eliminated (which must happen if the skin has lost that energy, which exercise of the body and cold ablutions can alone support), what becomes of the superfluous juices thus retained in the system? The answer is easy; they circulate through the internal organs and become the source of fevers, inflammations, dropsy, and all sorts of diseases. Medical men see these effects, but do not suppose them to have resulted from suppressed perspiration. Instead of attacking the skin, they assault the stomach and bowels, weaken the digestive organs, and by that means create disease; whilst water, on the contrary, is a remedy, possessing at once dissolving and strengthening properties, which would seem to neutralise each other, but that we have daily evidence to the contrary.

Herein lies the great secret of hydropathy: by its modes of application, morbid humours are drawn to the surface and eliminated, the body is cooled, and the skin put into a state to perform its indispensable duty. In internal inflammations, the morbid heat from the internal skin or mucous membrane is drawn off by the application of cold and irritation to the surface, and the disease subdued without charging the stomach with anything but pure spring water, which in contradistinction to drugs, produces the most salubrious effects.

The following extract shows that the skin is the great drain through which matters injurious to the system, and superfluous heat are drawn off and accounts for hydropathy being so universal a remedy.

A Practical Treatise on Healthy Skin, by Erasmus Wilson, *1 Vol. 1845.*
—Extract.

"The structure of the skin and the diseases to which it is liable, have latterly received from many of the medical profession considerable attention. The skin is that soft and pliant membrane which invests the whole of the external surface of the body, as also the interior which is called mucous membrane.

"The construction of these two membranes may easily inform us, without having recourse to fanciful hypotheses, how disease, affecting any part of this membrane, either internally or externally, may pass to any other part and affect the whole; and thus how a faulty digestion in a lady, a disease of the investing or mucous membrane of the stomach, may show itself in eruptions on the face. We see at once, too, how it happens that, calling into more active action the shower bath and flesh brush, dyspepsia may be avoided or cured. It serves also to explain the circumstance noticed by Fourcroy and Vauquelin, that the skin, with all its products, 'is capable of supplying the office of the kidneys,' and carrying off, as we know it to imbibe nourishment, the indispensable excretions for which the proper organs may be deficient.

"In explanation of this circumstance, we must remark, that the skin, internal or external, in which terminate all the arteries and commence the veins, in which too, the nerves of sensation commence, and the nerves of volition terminate, not only envelopes the whole body internally and externally, but is also the secretory organ of every part, and the immediate means of communication with the external world.

"The skin is the organ of contact with the external world, and the means of making us acquainted with every part of the universe. The senses of touch, of hearing, of smell, of taste, are all exercised by the skin.

"By the vessels terminating in the skin, or of which it is formed, all the phenomena of nutrition, and decay of appetite, and sensation, health and disease are produced.

"Whatever may be the climate or temperature in which the body is placed, it is kept at nearly one uniform and vital heat by the varying and adapting operations of the skin.

"The skin is the organ by which electricity is conducted into and out of the body.

"Its functions are, in short, proportioned to its vastness; and as it envelopes every part, so manifold are its purposes.

"The structure of the skin is highly curious; it consists of two layers; the one horny and insensible, guarding from injury; the other highly sensitive, the universal organ of feeling, which lies beneath; the latter feels, but the former dulls the impression.

"The following will show how, by the perspiratory organs, excess of water is removed from the blood, and the uniform temperature of the body preserved.

"Taken separately, the little perspiratory tube with its appended gland, is calculated to awaken in the mind very little idea of the importance of the system to which it belongs; but when the vast number of similar organs composing this system are considered, we are led to form some notion, however imperfect, of their probable influence in the health and comfort of the individual; the reality surpasses imagination and almost belief.

"The perspiratory pores on the palm of the hand, are found to be 3,528 in a square inch; now each of these pores being the aperture of a little tube of about a quarter of an inch long, it follows that in a square inch of skin on the palm of the hand, there exists a length of tube equal to 882 inches, or 73½ feet. Such a *drainage* as 73 feet in every square inch of skin, assuming this to be the average for the whole body, is something wonderful; and the thought naturally intrudes itself, What if this *drainage were obstructed? Could we need a stronger argument for enforcing the necessity of attention to the skin?* On the pulps of the finger, where the ridges of the sensitive layer of the true skin are somewhat finer than the palm of the hand and on the heel, where the ridges are coarser, the number of pores on the square inch was 2,268, and the length of tube 567 inches, or 47 feet. To obtain an estimate of the length of tube of the perspiratory system of the whole surface of the body, I think," says Dr. Wilson, "that 2,800 might be taken as a fair average of the number of pores in the square inch, and 700 consequently of the number of inches in length. Now the number of square inches of surface in a man of ordinary height and bulk is 2,500, the number of pores therefore, 7,000,000, and the number of inches of perspiratory tube 1,750,000, that is 145,833 feet, or 48,000 yards, or nearly 28 miles.

"This is only a specimen of the extraordinary structure.

"Besides the perspiratory vessels, the skin is provided with vessels for secreting an oily substance, which is of a different nature at different parts of the body; with vessels to repair abrasion and provide for its growth, and carry off its decayed parts; with nerves and blood-vessels that are probably as numerous and extensive as the perspiratory vessels.

"It must at the same time be remembered, that the interior skin or mucous membrane, is provided with equally numerous and complicated vessels, to answer some analogous purposes. The whole of them may be affected by applications to the external skin."

Dr. Wilson has, in his work, introduced some equally curious and instructive passages, as to the formation and uses of the oil-glands, the structure and functions of the hair, the influence of diet and clothing, and the effect of exercise and cleanliness on the health of this extensive organ.

V.—Is Hydropathy a Panacea? and what Complaints are curable by it?

Dr. Rauss, author of a work on hydropathy which passed through several editions, says, "It is almost impossible for any one to die of an acute disease, in whom reaction can be produced, and who from the commencement is treated Hydropathically.

"Those unacquainted with this treatment will naturally doubt its wonderful power; and the physician, when he reflects upon the number of patients who in acute diseases have perished under his hands, will no doubt treat it with derision; nevertheless," says the Doctor, "as I am not advancing a doctrine that may be controverted, *I here publicly make known that I am ready, by deeds as well as words, to prove all that I have stated.*" "To state," adds the Doctor, "$1" The cure of all acute diseases, of whatever nature or kind, with these exceptions, is to Priessnitz merely child's play; in no instance of nervous fevers or inflammations, in any stage, was he ever known to lose a patient; and what is worthy of remark in acute cases, a cure is effected in a few days without the subsequent debility which results from other treatment. Whilst I was at Gräfenberg, all descriptions of acute attacks came under my immediate notice, and I assert, without fear of contradiction, that they were all cured, with but one exception,—and that a highly valued friend of my own, a medical man, who was attacked with inflammation of the lungs. The doctor, who was advanced in life, retained his old prejudices, and consequently refused to submit to the treatment until too late. Confident in the power of Hydropathy for the last six years, whenever occasions offered (and they were not few during my sojourn in Ireland), I applied the treatment with invariable success. A case of inflammation of the mucous membrane is worthy of notice. One M. D. declared his belief that the patient would not live two hours; the other, that he could not exist until the evening. On the application of the wet sheet and tepid bath, the resuscitation of the man was as by miracle. In a case of diarrhoea, the rubbing sheet and its bath acted to the astonishment of the family. A young man had been under medical treatment for diarrhoea for a month, when he could not sleep more than a quarter of an hour at a time. He abandoned drugs, and was cured by hydropathy in three days. Dr. Engel of Vienna, and many other writers on the subject, are quite of the same opinion as Dr. Rauss as regards acute disease. This mode of treatment is efficacious in chronic diseases accompanied by atony; in all nervous affections, spasms, pains of which medicine will not discover the cause; in cases of obstruction of the bowels, and all the systematic evils which arise from them, such as indigestion, hypochondria, piles, jaundice, &c; in gout, rheumatism, scrofula, and most diseases affecting women; in fact, it is successful in a number of complaints altogether beyond the reach of medicine. I have had frequent occasions for admiring the result of the treatment in cases of ague, nervous, typhus, putrid, and scarlet fevers; but its most signal triumphs are obtained over those serious derangements of the system produced by the abuse of drugs, or when consumptions are produced by iodine, arsenic, or the consequences of mercury, tartar emetic, or other dangerous medicaments, have manifested themselves."

It may be stated without the fear of contradiction (not a word has been written to the contrary), that in small-pox, scarlatina, measles, croup, and all the complaints incidental to children; in fevers, inflammations, cholera, cholic, dysentery, diarrhoea, and, in fact, all acute diseases, hydropathy competently administered is omnipotent; and that in chronic complaints it effects more than can be obtained by any other means. The question is frequently put, "Will hydropathy cure all complaints?" I answer it is no catholicon, no panacea; nor is any cure for all diseases to be found.

> "As man, perhaps, the moment of his birth,
> Receives the lurking principle of death,
> The young disease that must subdue at length,
> Grows with his growth and strengthens with his strength."

Thus Pope viewed it, and thus it must be viewed by all who think on the subject. What the advocates of hydropathy assert is, that sudden fevers, of whatever nature they may be, diarrhoea, dysentery, cholera, English or Asiatic, in fact, all complaints that are termed acute, when the vital energies can be roused are sure of being cured; and that in old-standing complaints, usually denominated chronic, the water cure will do all that can be done by drugs, and that it is all-powerful over many complaints which are beyond the reach of all pharmaceutical remedies.

VI.—Is Hydropathy new? Why is it not generally adopted?

It is frequently said, by way of detracting from the merits of the Water-cure, that it is not new, that ages buried in the past have been witnesses to its merits. To this it may be replied, its advocates admit that the application of water to the cure of disease is as old as the hills;—but let me ask, breathes there a man who can point to the page, or call the dirty manuscript, from cavern or chest, wherein lies hid the present process of Hydropathy's main arms, the wet sheet, sweating process, the douche, etc.? Where shall we find the sage of ancient or modern times, buried in herbalistic lore and practice, that ever succeeded so completely in the cure of diseases, by thrusting nothing upon his patient's stomachic organs but pure unadulterated water, as Priessnitz? We seek not to prove its novelty, but its utility.

It has been shewn that water as a curative agent, has been known from the remotest period; but its means of application were insufficient. In the days of Pliny, it agitated the Roman world. In the sixteenth century, great efforts were made in our own country to introduce it into practice, and again more lately, the subject was agitated, but it did not advance. Thus it has been with all great discoveries—witness Steam. Le Caus, who discovered its powers two hundred years ago, was consigned to a mad-house. The French Academy of Science denounced Fulton's discovery as a chimera and absurd, as it did Hydropathy a few years since. Others, anxious for the existence of a hidden treasure, were ever in search of it, each step conducted slowly nearer the goal; but a Watt, was required to give full and vigorous development to its powers. Thus, it has been with water, which, unaided by its present manifold modes of application, was nearly as ungovernable as the steam without the engine.

All nations recognised and many partially profited by the healing properties of water; but the genius of a Priessnitz was required to explore its capabilities and resources, and, by reducing them to a science, confer an inestimable boon on mankind and scatter to the winds the accumulated fallacies of ages.

If all these effects which we have shown, are to be produced by Hydropathic appliances, is it not evident there is something to be learnt? An acquaintance with its details, its *modus operandi*, can only be acquired by study and experience, as Lady Morgan says, "knowledge is a fruit which no longer grows upon trees; on the contrary, it partakes more of the nature of the truffle, and must be dug for by those who are desirous of tasting it."[2]

A Medical Education does not necessarily assist in the knowledge of Hydropathy; on the contrary, it acts as barrier to the acquirement of a perfect insight into it. Hydropathy and Allopathy in their practice are like the poles asunder.

The question is frequently mooted, if Hydropathy is so harmless and yet so certain in its operations, how is it that the medical professors, whose object is to relieve their fellow-men, and prolong their lives, do not take it up? To this it might be answered, "It is a difficult thing to force any to believe the evidence of their own senses, if their instincts or their interests (which are one and the same) happen to point another way."

"In the practice of Medicine, as in every thing else, there are vested interests, those in the receipt of large sums of money are content with things as they are, those in more limited practice have not the courage to enter upon anything new, however persuaded of its utility. Others are deterred by the fear of being considered Quacks, or losing cast[e] with their brother practitioners, and all see, that, in the ordinary occurrences of life the application of Hydropathy is so simple, that were it generally practised, nine tenths of the faculty would have to throw up their briefs. A writer in Chamber's Journal justly observes,—"If the subject be new and startling, and still more so, if any interest or prejudice be disturbed by it, the clearest demonstration on earth is of no avail."

Since the education of medical men (totally at variance as it is with all the principles of the Water-cure), gives them no advantage whatever over a non-medical man in judging of what is, or what is not a fit case for Hydropathy; or, in prescribing its practice, any opinion from the faculty, opposed as their interest, and prejudices are to it, ought to be received for as much as it is worth, and no more. One thinks Hydropathy available in gout —another doubts that, but believes it to be good in fevers or inflammations —a third would not hesitate to apply it in dysentery or diarrhœa—a fourth, for a cold—and so on through the whole category of disease; but, with the gravity of true sons of Aesculapius, to their own patients they recommend caution, which at once deters them from trying it. When these practitioners are asked, how they arrived at the conclusion, that the complaints they name may be cured by this treatment, their reasons are entirely speculative; and when pressed as to why they do not apply it, inasmuch as they admit it to be good, they argue the impossibility of contending with public prejudices.

Might we not ask, who are the authors of this state of things? Few people think for themselves, either in Law, Physic, or Divinity. As long as incomes from one thousand to thirty thousand pounds a year (and that there are the latter is proved by the returns of the Income Tax), are made by members of the profession, no reform with their consent can be expected. At one period, after the amputation of a limb, bleeding was staunched by the application of boiling pitch. Paré deprecated this treatment, and recommended the taking up arteries, as is now done. He was treated with derision: "What" said the old practitioner, "would you hang the life of a man upon a thread?" When Harvey propounded his theory, he lost caste with his brethren, and a medical writer doubts if any practitioner of the period, who had passed forty years, believed in the circulation of the blood.

Jenner, to secure himself from the fury of a mob, sought refuge in the house of Colonel Wilson; and there is still a minute in the books of the Foundling Hospital, the first public establishment that adopted Vaccination, stating that as its application could not be entrusted to the faculty, the Committee recommended that the operation of vaccination should be performed by the Clergy.

Lady Mary Wortley Montague was so persecuted, that she always regretted having introduced inoculation into the country.

VII.—THE LANCET.

The use of the Lancet is a subject that ought to interest every friend to humanity in an especial manner. By this, our mortal foe, more have fallen than by the sword. The use of one is as unjustifiable as the other. "Blood is the life," this is the language of holy writ; he who sheds that, deprives us of a part of our existence.

"The use of the Lancet," says Dr. Dickson, "was the invention of an unenlightened, possibly a sanguinary age; and its continued use says but little for the after-discoveries of ages, or for the boasted progress of medical science.

"Will the men who thus lovingly pour out the blood, dispute its importance in the animal economy? Will they deny that it forms the basis of the solids, —that when the body has been wasted by long diseases, it is by the blood only it can recover its healthy volume and appearance?

"Misguided by theory, man, presumptuous man, has dared to divide what God, as a part of creation, has united; to open what the Eternal, in the wisdom of his omniscience made entire.

"It is on the face of it a most unnatural proceeding. How can you withdraw blood from one organ without depriving every other of the material of its healthy state?

"The first resource of the surgeon is the lancet. The first thing he thinks of, when called to an accident, is how he can most quickly open the flood-gates of the heart, to pour out the stream of an already enfeebled existence."

Capt. Owen, in detailing the mortality which took place among his people on the coast of Africa, by yellow fever, says, "he had not one instance of perfect recovery after a liberal application of the lancet. And in the subsequent report of the Select Committee on the Western Coast of Africa, there occurs the following passage. "The bleeding system has fortunately gone out of fashion; and the frightful mortality that attended its practice, is now no longer known on board our ships."

"Let the reader," says Dr. Gibbs, in his letters from Gräfenberg, "enter the crowded hospitals in England or the Continent, and see how mercilessly the lancet, the leech, and cupping-glass are employed in the diseases of the poor. Look at the pale and ghastly faces of the inmates."

Among the numerous diseases which bleeding can produce, Darwin says, a paroxysm of gout is liable to recur. John Hunter mentions lock-jaw and dropsy; Travers, blindness and palsy; Marshall Hall, mania; Blundell, dysentery; Broussais, fever and convulsion. "When an animal loses a considerable quantity of blood," says John Hunter, "the heart increases in frequency of strokes, as also in its violence." Yet these are the indications for which professors bleed. Magendie mentions *pneumonia* as having been produced by it; and further tells us, that he has witnessed among its effects "the entire train of inflammatory phenomena;" and mark, he adds the extraordinary fact, "that this inflammation will have been produced by the very agent chiefly used to combat it." We read in scripture, "He that sheddeth man's blood, by man shall his blood be shed." It has ever been supposed, that this applied to the assassin; but holy writ is deeper than this! and no doubt the time will come, when one man will no more think of bleeding another, than he would of committing any other act that should expose him to public ignominy.

The operation of blood-letting is so associated in the minds of most men with the practice of physic, that when a sensible German physician, some time ago, petitioned the king of Prussia to make the employment of the lancet penal, he was laughed at from one end of Europe to the other.

"The imputation of novelty," says Locke, "is a terrible charge against those who judge of men's heads as they do of their perukes, by the *fashion*; and can allow none to be right, but the received doctrine." Thus Hydropathy, like many other valuable discoveries, and even Christianity itself, must wait its time; a circumstance much to be lamented—because all that is sought by bleeding is effected without this soul-harrowing process. Let such as doubt the fact, go to Gräfenberg, there they will learn that during the whole course of Mr. Priessnitz's practice, not a single drop of human blood has been spilt; and yet all diseases for which the lancet is applied are hourly relieved. This is a fact so notorious, that no pen has ever been raised to deny it; so long as interest governs prejudice, practitioners may continue their destructive practice with impunity; but where are the feelings? As observed by a writer, "what a long dream of false security have mankind been dreaming! They have laid themselves down on the laps of their medical Mentors, they have slept a long sleep; while these, like the fabled vampire of the poet, taking advantage of a dark night of barbarism and ignorance, have thought it no sin to rob them of their life's blood, during the profoundness of their slumber."

Dr. Kitto, in his clever work on consumption says;—"On the subject of bleeding, purgatives, mercury, and a low course of diet, I shall have occasion to show, in the course of my observations, that these agents are not only unnecessary, but actually mischievous, particularly bleeding, which has proved more fatal than the pestilence or the sword. Nature is our best and surest guide; and if we would follow only her admonitions, we should not so frequently have to witness the impotence of our efforts to alleviate suffering; or to mourn the unfortunate results of cases, which, despite the boasted improvements in the healing art, but too frequently terminate in the grave."

VIII.—AUTHORITIES IN SUPPORT OF WATER AS A CURATIVE AGENT.

Thales, like Homer, looked upon water as the principle of every thing. The Spartans bathed their children as soon as born in cold water; and the men of Sparta, both old and young, bathed at all seasons of the year in the Eurotas, to harden their flesh and strengthen their bodies.

Pindar, in one of his Olympic Odes, says, "The best thing is water, and the next gold."

There was a Greek proverb to the effect that the water of the sea cured all ills.

Pythagoras recommended the use of cold baths strongly to his disciples, to fortify both body and mind.

Hippocrates, the father of medicine, who added friction to cold bathing, was accustomed to use cold water in his treatment of the most serious illnesses. It was Hippocrates who first observed that warm water chilled, whilst cold water warmed.

The Macedonians considered warm water to be enervating; and their women, after accouchement, were washed with cold water.

Virgil called the ancient inhabitants of Italy, a race of men hard and austere, who immersed their newly-born children in the rivers, and accustomed them to cold water.

Pliny, in speaking of A. Musa, who cured Horace by means of cold water, said that he put an end to confused drugs; and he also alludes to a certain Charmes, who made a sensation at Rome by the cures he effected with cold water. On being asked what he thought drugs were sent for, he said, "he could not imagine, except that men might destroy themselves with them when they were tired of living."

Celsus, called the Cicero of doctors, employed water for complaints of the head and stomach.

Galen, in the second century, recommended cold bathing to the healthy, as well as to patients labouring under the attacks of fever.

Charlemagne, aware of the salubrity of cold bathing, encouraged the use of it throughout his empire, and introduced swimming as an amusement at his court.

Michael Savonarola, an Italian doctor, in 1462, recommended cold water in gout, ophthalmia, and hæmorrhages.

Cardanus, of Pavia, 1575, complains that the doctors in his time made so little use of cold water in the curing of gout.

Van der Heyden, a doctor at Ghent, in a work published in 1624, states that during an epidemic dysentery, he cured many hundreds of persons with cold water, and that during a long practice of fifty years, the best cures he ever made were effected with cold water.

Short, an English doctor, 1656, states that he had cured the dropsy and the bite of mad dogs with cold water.

Dr. Sir John Floyer published a work, called "the Psychrolusic," in 1702, showing how fevers were to be cured with water. From that period to 1722, his work went through six editions in London.

Dr. Hancock, in 1722, published an anti-fever treatise upon the use of cold water, which went through seven editions in one year.

Dr. Currie of Liverpool, who published a work in 1797, on the use of water, introduced that element extensively in his practice with astounding results.

Tissot, in his "Advice to the People," published in Paris, 1770, shows the importance of cold water.

Hoffman, the famous German doctor, says that if there existed anything in the world that could be called a panacea, it was pure water: first, because that element would disagree with nobody; secondly, because it is the best preservative against disease; thirdly, because it would cure agues and chronic complaints; fourthly because it responded to all indications.

Hahn, who was born in Silesia, in 1714, wrote an excellent work upon the curative agency of water in all complaints, a copy was lately found upon a book-stall, and purchased by Professor Oertel, for little more than one penny, and has been re-published; it is interesting to all who regard with attention that great moral change which the Water-cure is calculated to effect.

In Dr. Hahn's work, it is stated that Pater Bernardo, a Capuchin monk from Sicily, went in the year 1724 to Malta, and there made some most astonishing water-cures, the fame of which spread throughout Europe: he used iced water internally and externally, and allowed his patients to eat but very little. He made a proposition that the doctors should take 100 patients, and said if they, by their mode of treating them, could cure forty, then would he undertake to cure sixty more easily and securely, and in a shorter time. His remedy of iced water, was just as effectual in winter as in summer. A case is cited of a man, ninety-two years of age, who was at the point of death from the virulence of a fever, and was cured with cold water only.

Evan Hahnemann, father of Homeopathy, in a work published at Leipsic, 1784, recommends fresh water, without which, he says, ulcers of any long standing cannot be cured, and adds, if there be any general remedy for disease, "it is water."

The Rev. John Wesley, A.M., published a work in 1747 (about a century ago), which went through thirty-four editions, called "Primitive Physic, or an Easy and Natural Method of Curing most Diseases."

After deprecating the manner in which drugs were imposed upon mankind, the mysteries with which the science of medicine is surrounded, and the interested conduct of medical men, the Rev. gentleman proceeds to shew, that he was fully aware of the healing powers of water; and from the long list which he has given, and which follows, it will be evident that he thought water capable of curing almost every disease to which human nature is exposed. He writes:—

"The common method of compounding and decompounding medicines, can never be reconciled to common sense. Experience shews, that one thing will cure most disorders, at least as well as twenty put together. Then why do you add the other nineteen? Only to swell the apothecary's bill! nay, possibly on purpose to prolong the distemper, that the doctor and he may divide the spoil.

"How often, by thus compounding medicines of opposite qualities, is the virtue of both utterly destroyed?

"Nay, how often do those joined together destroy life, which singly they might have preserved?

"This occasioned that caution of the great Boerhaave, against mixing things without evident necessity, and without full proof of the effect they will produce when joined together, as well as of that they produce when asunder; seeing (as he observes) that several things which taken separately are safe and powerful medicines, when compounded not only lose their former power, but compose a strong and deadly poison."

In recommending to his followers the use of water, Mr. Wesley proceeds to state, *"that cold bathing cures young children of the following complaints:* —

Convulsions, coughs, gravel	Pimples and scabs
Inflammations of ears, navel and mouth	Suppression of urine
Rickets	Vomiting
Cutaneous inflammations	Want of sleep

"Water," he further adds, "frequently cures every nervous[3] and every paralytic disorder. In particular:—

Asthma	Leprosy (old)
Agues of every sort	Lethargy
Atrophy	Loss of speech, taste, appetite, smell
Blindness	Nephritic pains
Cancer	Palpitation of the heart
Coagulated blood of bruises	Pain in the back, joints, stomach
Chin cough	Rheumatism
Consumption	Rickets
Convulsions	Rupture
Coughs	Suffocations
Complication of distempers	Surfeits at the beginning
Convulsive pains	Sciatica
Deafness	Scorbutic pains
Dropsy	Swelling in the joints
Epilepsy	Stone in the kidneys
Violent fever	Torpor of the limbs, even when the use of them is lost
Gout (running)	Tetanus
Hectic fevers	Tympany
Hysteric pains	Vertigo
Incubus	St. Vitus' dance
Inflammations	Vigilia
Involuntary stool or urine	Varicose ulcers
Lameness	The Whites

"Water prevents the growth of hereditary

Apoplexies	King's evil
Asthmas	Melancholy
Blindness	Palsies
Consumptions	Rheumatism
Deafness	Stone
Gout	

"Water drinking water generally prevents

Apoplexies	Madness
Asthma	Palsies

Convulsions	Stone
Gout	Trembling.
Hysteric fits	

"To this children should be used from their cradles."

We then find the following prescriptions:—

"*For Asthma.*—Take a pint of cold water every morning, washing the head in cold water immediately after, and using the cold bath.

"*Rickets in Children.*—Dip them in cold water every morning.

"*To prevent apoplexy.*—Use the cold bath and drink only cold water.

"*Ague.*—Go into a cold bath just before the cold.

"*Cancer in the breast.*—Use the cold bath. This has cured many. This cured Mrs. Bates, of Leicestershire, of a cancer in her breast, a consumption, a sciatica, and rheumatism, which she had had nearly twenty years.

N.B. Generally where cold bathing is necessary to cure disease, water-drinking is so, to prevent a relapse.

"*Hysteric colic.*—Mrs. Watts, by using the cold bath two and twenty times in a month, was entirely cured of an hysteric colic, fits, and convulsive motions, continual sweatings and vomitings, wandering pains in her limbs and head, and total loss of appetite.

"*To prevent the ill effects of cold.*—The moment a person gets into a house, with his hands and feet quite chilled, let him put them into a vessel of water, as cold as can be got, and hold them there until they begin to glow, which they will do in a minute or two. This method likewise effectually prevents chilblains.

"*Consumption.*—Cold bathing has cured many deep consumptions.

"*Convulsions.*—Use the cold bath."

And so on. In this valuable little work, from which are the above extracts, confirmative of the value I set upon cold water, Mr. Wesley prescribes the use of water for almost every complaint.

Slade, in his "Records of the East," very judiciously remarks, with reference to the Turks, that "notwithstanding their ignorance of medical science, added to the extreme irregularity of their living, both as regards diet and exercise, one day dining off cheese and cucumbers, another day feeding on ten greasy dishes; one month riding twelve hours daily, another month never stirring off the sofa; smoking always, and drinking coffee to excess; occasionally getting drunk, besides other intemperances—combining, in short, all that our writers on the subject designate injurious to health—the Turks enjoy particularly good health: and this anomaly is owing to two causes; first, the religious necessity of washing their arms and feet and necks, from three to five times a day, always with cold water, generally at the fountains before the mosques, by which practice they become protected against catarrhal affections; second, by their constant use of the vapour bath, by which the humours that collect in the human frame, no doctors know how or why, occasioning a long list of disorders, are carried off by the pores of the skin. Gout, rheumatism, head-ache, consumption, are unknown in Turkey, thanks to the great physicians, vapour bath and cold bath! No art has been so much vitiated in Europe, by theories, as the art of preserving health. Its professors, however, are beginning to recur to first principles; and when bathing shall be properly appreciated, three-fourths of the druggists will be obliged to close their shops."

The question here arises: how is it that with so much evidence in favour of water, it has never been brought into general use? Many reasons might be assigned, but the principal one is, that until the present day no system of treatment has ever been based on scientific principles. It was in embryo, and, like Steam, wanted its time for development. If people studied their health as they do their interest, they would at least enquire into this, the best means of preserving it.

But in our present state of civilisation, nature is known by name only. None save those reduced to the last stage of poverty ever satisfy their thirst with water! Men, women, and children, rich and poor, old and young, all avoid water—perhaps because it costs nothing (for, in our artificial life, we are led to esteem things according to their venal price), and, like air and sun, is shared in common with our poorer fellow-kind.

The Germans are water-drinkers, but the English have a distaste for it; few ever drank half a pint undiluted at one time, in their lives, imagining that water will cause inconvenience, whilst in the course of the day, they think nothing of drinking wine, soda water, brandy and water, and tea, to a great extent, all of which are injurious. A lady of my acquaintance carries her distaste for water so far as to ruin the health of her children by it. For some time the eldest, about four years old, had been sickly: when at Rome, the mother consulted a medical man, who said that the child wanted nothing but water, which was given it, and the child got well immediately. I met the same family at Kissingen, when at a spring the nursery-maid asked me if she might give the child water, saying the children were always asking for it, but her mistress did not like them to drink water alone. "Certainly," I replied, "give her as much as she chooses to drink."

In addition to cold water, fresh air and exercise are most important means of health. They are especially useful in giving life and activity to the skin, which seldom meets with proper attention, people generally not being aware of the evil consequences attending their neglect of that most important organ of the human frame.

By protecting the skin from the air, we concentrate on it the heat that is ever exhaling from the body, and thus complete what warm baths, spirituous liquors, want of exercise, close rooms, and heavy nourishment, have begun. We do not perceive that by keeping the body warm, we weaken the skin, which becomes so sensitive to external changes, that we are incessantly obliged to augment the thickness and number of its coverings. At last, a time comes when nothing more can be added to the clothing already too heavy. Then weak and irritable persons, whose numbers—our erroneous system daily augments!—remain at home, not aware of the innumerable inconveniences to which such a resolution exposes them, and not knowing that the habitual washing of the body in cold water, would enable them to leave their heated apartments, abandon flannel, and expose themselves, without the slightest danger, to the healthy effects of fresh air.

It is the enervating softness and delicacy of modern customs, which present the greatest obstacle to the use of cold water. Man looks for agreeable impressions, and avoids whatever does not produce them. But with a little courage, he would discover that the inconvenience of a more rigorous and simple mode of life was but momentary, and when he had found his health of mind and body improved by it, it would soon become agreeable, whilst from luxurious sloth ensue enervation and disgust. Being unable to change the nature of the elements, we should harden our bodies, familiarise ourselves with the inclemency of the seasons, and turn them to the benefit of our health. It is in vain that the man whose fortune permits him to change the climate, looks for a milder sky; if his effeminacy accompanies him, he will be like a lady of whom Priessnitz speaks, who near the fire was cold. A warmer air would enervate his skin more and more; and then he would be as sensitive to cold, even in a Neapolitan climate, as, with a hardened body, he would be at his ease in the hut of an Esquimaux.

Another obstacle to the external use of cold water, is the false belief that colds, which are the sources of much illness, result from it. People cannot understand that a cold bath, followed by suitable exercise, warms the feet and the body, and that there is *no* surer preservative from cold.

The same incredulity is affected with regard to the revulsive effect of the cold foot-bath; nevertheless nothing is better proved than its efficiency in relieving the head. Every one knows that, after having washed the face and hands in cold water, an agreeable warmth ensues, which is not the result of warm water. That after any part of the body has been exposed to cold, rain, or snow, it becomes hot; and that the reverse is the case after the use of warm water; which accounts for people in Summer feeling cool after a warm bath.

When we wash the body with cold water, we should do it quickly, lose no time in dressing, and afterwards take exercise. Washing should be avoided when the parties are cold, because then the re-action or re-production of heat is slower. These precautions would prevent the most delicate persons from taking cold, though not in the habit of using cold water.

Professor Oertel was the first to publish to the world the astonishing cures which were effected at Gräfenberg; and he was followed by Brand, Kroeber, Kurtsz, Doering, Harnish, and a host of others, whose writings contributed to establish the reputation of Priessnitz, who by means of the various forms in which he administers water, attacks all diseases susceptible of cure, and very frequently establishes the health of those who have been declared incurable.

IX.—ABLUTIONS.

There can be no doubt, if the public were in the habit of using cold ablutions every morning, their health would be improved, and the number of consumptive cases much diminished.

There are many ways of using ablutions, according to the health and strength of the parties.

Strong people ought to go into a cold bath the moment they get out of bed; then rub themselves well for three or four minutes. If not in their usual health, the bath should be protracted, and more friction used.

Another or general mode is to have a washing tub, water only two or three inches deep, put a towel into the water, leave the bed quite warm, step into the tub, take up the towel with as much water as possible, and squeeze it over the head and shoulders several times, rub the body well with the towel, then sit down in the tub, and with wet hands rub the abdomen, etc., for a minute or two.

Delicate persons may be washed all over with wet towels; sometimes it is desirable to wash first with tepid water, then with cold.

Where there is a great whiteness of skin, which indicates a want of circulation, or parties feel themselves indisposed, dripping sheets are prescribed; the friction here used arouses the vital energies, and in general produces a most refreshing feeling throughout the system.

Priessnitz never prescribes cold immersion till the body be prepared for it. When patients have been desirous of bathing in a river, he has always opposed it; saying, "Bathing excites nervous sensibility; too much bathing excites the system to an injurious extent." The various baths resorted to in hydropathy, are to effect an object, and as such are medically applied. Sea bathing for some constitutions is remarkably wholesome, but to others it is injurious.

X.—Use of Cold Water for Drinking and Injections.

Dr. Arbuthnot, in his work on aliments, says that "Water is the chief ingredient in the animal fluids and solids; for a dry bone distilled, affords a great quantity of insipid water: therefore, water seems to be the proper drink for every animal." Berzelius, the great Swedish chemist, proved the truth of Dr. Arbuthnot's observations, by distilling the entire corpse of a moderate sized man down to water, with the exception of eight pounds.

And Milton has expressed his concurrence with those authorities in eloquent language, when speaking of Samson:—

> "O madness! to think use of strongest wines,
> And strongest drink, our chief support of health,
> When, God, with these forbidden, made choice to rear
> His mighty champion, strong above compare,
> Whose drink was only from *the limpid brook*."

About twelve ordinary size tumblers of water a day are generally drunk whilst under the treatment; instances occur where that number is increased to twenty, and even thirty glasses, but such are very rare.

At the beginning it is difficult to drink so much water; but by degrees we become accustomed to it. All the operations of the cure lead to the elimination of heat, which naturally causes thirst. Some persons on first drinking water feel sick, or have diarrhoea, which proves that the stomach is not in a healthy state. In this case, instead of discontinuing the drinking of water, the quantity is increased. When pain in the stomach comes from its being overcharged by food, water, in large quantities is recommended to be persevered in until relief is obtained.

We know that emetics produce this effect, but such remedies weaken the stomach—while water has the contrary tendency.

Cold water, as a beverage, fortifies the stomach and intestines, by clearing them of the bad juices they contain: favours the generation of new juices, and mixes with the blood by absorption. It spreads itself quickly through all the organs, attenuates, purifies, and dissolves the sharp or thick humours, and discharges them by means of perspiration and urine. Considered as a dietetic for slight indispositions, bad digestions, and generally in all cases of disease for which the faculty recommend aperients or mineral waters, it cannot be too highly appreciated. In the morning, after a cold ablution, whilst taking exercise, drink a few tumblers of water, and conclude every meal with a tumbler of water. It will have the same effect as a purgative or mineral water, without, like them, weakening the digestive organs. All persons may drink cold water at all times of the day with impunity, if they are not inconvenienced by it. That taken before breakfast, during exercise, produces doubtless the best effects. It is above all after sweating that drinking cold water produces an expectoration of phlegm. Water may be drunk after breakfast, but not so as to overcharge the stomach. During dinner the aliments should be moistened by some glasses of water, then the stomach must be left to repose; some hours afterwards again water may be drunk until supper-time. Drinking after supper is no less useful; but it may break the rest, by causing an invalid to rise often in the night. After drinking, exercise is indispensable, it stimulates the action of the water, and accelerates a cure. When in exercise, though in a perspiration, water may be drunk in any quantities. Water ought always to be drawn fresh from the spring, and drunk as cold as possible. The decanters which contain it ought to have stoppers, to preserve it cold and fresh. After every operation in the cure, a glass of water should be drunk; and it should be given in small quantities when in the sweating process. I know a gentleman who has all his life been a free-liver, and who, notwithstanding, is in good health, which he attributes entirely to drinking a couple of tumblers of water the last thing at night and first thing in the morning.

Under the denomination of injections, we principally understand clysters. When the patient is not in the habit of using them with cold water, they must not at first be applied for longer than two minutes; but by degrees the intestines become accustomed to the water, which is often absorbed like that introduced into the stomach. When necessary, a second injection is repeated immediately after the expulsion of the first.[4] Cold injections are used for constipation and diarrhoea, two diseases diametrically opposite, but which arise from the same cause, the weakness of the intestines. Thus the contradiction is only in appearance, the great object of injections being to establish the tone of these organs, and regulate their functions. Injections ought to be aided by the use of cold water in other ways.

There are also other injections in use at Gräfenberg, such as for the ears, nostrils, and genitals. Particular syringes are used for these purposes.

XI.—THE COLD BATH.

The cold plunge-bath should be sufficiently deep for a man of ordinary height to plunge into, up to his arm-pits. The water aught[sic] to be continually renewed by a spring.

We have quoted many authorities to shew the advantages resulting from exposing the body to the action of cold water.

When cold baths disagree with us, it is because we are not in a state to use them, or we stay in too long.

When the body is overcharged with drugs or alcohol, when the juices are dried up, or when there is an apoplectic tendency, and when in other diseased conditions, the circulation is languid, cold plunge-baths must be used with great caution. Many suppose that all the patients in a hydropathic establishment, are indiscriminately ordered this sort of bath. In this they err, because many are never allowed their use, and others only after a long application of the rubbing sheet and tepid baths. Strong robust constitutions may take the plunge-bath at once; but in the Water-cure this is not allowed until the body is prepared for it, and then only for a short time; generally for three or four minutes. Priessnitz objects to persons staying long in the water: of course the objection applies to invalids. For those who bathe in the sea, or other water, he does not pretend to prescribe.

Every day's experience proves that the immersion of the body, covered with perspiration into cold water, is exempt from danger, provided the internal organs are in state of repose.

The risk which is incurred of catching cold on stripping and bathing in a river, in this case cannot apply, as the body heated by artificial means is at once immersed, whilst the bather often, injudiciously, waits until chilled before he enters the water.

If we walk fast, or a long distance, to the bath, it is requisite to repose a little to tranquillise the lungs; then before perspiration ceases, we ought to undress quietly, and either plunge head foremost into the water, or wet the head and chest previously, to prevent the blood mounting to those regions.

Whilst bathing, the head ought to be immersed several times. After the sweating or packing process, great care is to be observed in not exposing any part of the body to the air previous to entering the bath. The patient should keep in movement, rubbing himself well the whole time. This stimulates the skin and abates the cold.

The time for remaining in the bath, is governed by the coldness of the water, and the vital heat of the bather; a second sensation of cold is to be avoided, or re-action may be difficult.

On leaving the bath, the patient is covered with a dry sheet, upon which the attendant rubs, until the body presents a warm healthy glow. The invalid should then dress quickly, drink a glass or two of water, and walk out in the air to get warm; to effect this by the heat of stoves or beds would be acting in direct opposition to Hydropathic rules.

When irritation is excited during the cure, the cold bath is sometimes suspended and tepid baths resorted to. Every house ought to be supplied with a cold bath, as its habitual use by the members of the family would secure them against colds, influenza, etc.

Priessnitz says, "that the effect of going into cold water without being previously heated, and doing so in a state of perspiration, is like a blacksmith hammering upon cold, rather than hot iron. Cramp frequently attends the former, whilst a healthy reaction is always the result of the latter."

XII.—Is going into the Cold Bath in a State of Perspiration attended with Danger?

"The transition from a Vapour-bath to snow, or to a Cold-bath, has been practised by the Russians for time immemorial" with the most beneficial results,—"this," adds Dr. Johnson, "is conclusive, that there is no danger whatever in going into the Cold-bath while covered with perspiration; unless it can be proved that perspiration produced by hot vapour is a very different thing from perspiration produced by a blanket;" and, adds the learned doctor, in his valuable work on Hydropathy, which every one ought to read; "All physiological reasoning goes to prove, that it is safer to go into cold water when the temperature of the skin has been raised.

"If there be danger at all, it is going into cold water *without* raising the temperature of the body. It must be the temperature that is the question; for it cannot be of consequence whether the body be covered with grease called perspiration or hog's-lard. Re-action will most certainly be produced, and congestion as certainly prevented by going into the water when the body is warm. Profuse perspiration does not make the body hotter, in proportion to its profuseness, on the contrary, it is cooler than before, for perspiration is a cooling process.

"When perspiration is present, the body is never extremely hot. Checking perspiration is a chimerical danger; the oozing of perspiration subsides of itself, almost at the moment the means that produced it are withdrawn, and the perspiration on the body is that which has been already produced, having now no connection with the body."

At Cork in Ireland, it was told me by one of the first brewers, that formerly his men, while in a state of perspiration, from pressing the grain out of the vats, frequently caught cold and died: at last they adopted the plan of going into cold water, whilst in that state; the result of which has been that they now never catch cold from their occupation, and are as healthy as other people.

XIII.—The Packing Sheet, and Sweating Process.

Take all the coverings off the bed, arrange the pillows, cover over the bed and pillows with a large thick blanket, then put a small sheet into a pail of fresh cold water; if to reduce fever, let it be wrung out less; if there is no fever, more; the drier the sheet, the sooner the re-action; spread this sheet so wrung out, on the blanket.

The patient extends himself, divested of every thing, upon the sheet, which should be brought over him as soon as possible. The blanket is now brought over the sheet, and the attendant tucks it in, beginning with the neck, as tightly as possible, so that his patient can hardly move hand or foot. Other blankets are then added, separately tucked in, and turned up at the feet. Half-a-dozen blankets are not too many; and to produce immediate heat, a feather bed is superadded, leaving the head free. It is astonishing what an amount of covering one may support without inconvenience.

The great object is so to envelop the body as to exclude the air, and prevent evaporation, in order that its own heat may be concentrated upon itself.

In ordinary cases, the sheet is well wrung out, and covered up as before stated; but in cases of severe fever, the wet is only covered with a single dry one. In cases of very great delicacy, but not in fever, the sheet is put into tepid water instead of cold.

This has by some been called a general poultice, as it performs upon the whole body what a poultice or the bandages effect upon members of it. Dr. Alexander of Newcastle terms it a linen bath.

That wet linen should produce good and evil results appears paradoxical. Damp beds are said to lead to injurious consequences, whilst wet linen applied as a covering to the whole or parts of the body, produces the most happy effects.

Accustomed as Priessnitz is to witnessing none but the best results from the application of damp linen, he could not be persuaded that mischief arose even from lying in damp beds.

In the Hydropathic practice the body is so hermetically enclosed in the wet sheet, that not a particle of heat can escape or external air penetrate, by which means the exhalation is concentrated upon the body; this may be termed a linen bath or fomentation.

In the case of people being accidentally put into a damp bed, none of the above precautions are taken; there is no extra clothing, no binding about the neck to prevent the escape of caloric, and therefore to these causes must be attributed the mischief, if any ensue.

It is, however, a question, where mischief follows, whether one-twentieth part of the cases can be fairly attributed to the damp beds. It is highly probable that Priessnitz's surmise of its being the development of a disease lurking in the system which under the Water-cure might easily be met, is correct.

Wet sheets are resorted to in all fevers, and changed until the paroxysm is abated. In Typhus, the sheet is changed every ten minutes, and as often as forty or fifty times in a day.

As a general rule, Mr. Priessnitz told me, if unwell, without waiting to know the ailment—to take a packing-sheet, until warm, twice a day, followed by a tepid bath.

Packing-sheets may be persevered in for years in obstinate cases. The usual time employed in their application is until the body is warm, which will be from twenty-five to forty minutes. It is a great mistake to suppose the application of the sheet is to produce perspiration. If a genial heat pervades the body, it is all that is required, unless under peculiar circumstances, previous to immersion in either tepid or cold water.

The following anecdote, told me by Major Beavan, is adduced as corroborative evidence in favour of the use of wet linen to lower the temperature of the body. In 1821, the Major having to pass through extensive jungles to join his regiment in the East Indies, a distance of nearly 300 miles, caught a fever. When at the highest stage of the hot fit, it occurred to him that he might cool himself as they did wine and other liquids in that climate. He accordingly had himself wrapped up in a wet sheet for a quarter of an hour, when, finding himself relieved, he added a number of coverings, and fell into a most refreshing sleep of some hours. On awaking, he found mind, body, and appetite restored, all of which had been prostrated to an extreme degree for several days.

The packing-sheet is the greatest sedative known. It generally occurs that persons who, from pain or nervous excitement, have not slept for nights, doze off immediately on being enveloped in the wet sheet.

The packing-sheet brings morbific matter to the surface, and thereby relieves the capillaries. The ablution which follows acts as a tonic.

The relief afforded to the overcharged system through the pores, by the application of the packing-sheet, may be compared to the emptying of a bason with a sponge; each sheet absorbing a certain amount of morbific matter and superfluous animal heat, until the body is relieved.

In fevers generally, the fœtid odour of the sheet when withdrawn, is hardly to be endured; and in eruptive fevers, the inclination to scratch the body is allayed, and very little inconvenient sensation is felt either night or day.

In the morning, when fever is most felt, wet sheets and tepid baths allay it; and in the afternoon, any return of it is again subdued as before. The discovery of the wet sheet alone is sufficient to render the name of Priessnitz immortal.

But when, by these means, it would be difficult to produce perspiration, recourse is previously had to a dripping or rubbing-sheet, and then the patient is packed up; or the blanket is warmed before a fire, before the body is enveloped in it.

The sweating process, when used, is always succeeded by a tepid or cold bath, or a dripping-sheet: if a tepid bath, cold water is afterwards poured over the head and shoulders; but if a dripping-sheet, it is repeated until the body is cooled.

Every day's practice at Gräfenberg, and elsewhere, shews that no danger attends going into cold water in a heated state.

But Mr. Priessnitz, whether from having a different class of patients, or from the difficulty of getting servants to understand when the patient had perspired enough, or the conviction that the same or better results attend the packing sheet, we know not, has changed his practice, and no longer resorts so frequently to the sweating process. The following extract is from a letter received by the author from a gentleman who has been a long time at Gräfenberg.

"The object of all Hydropathic appliances may be shortly and intelligibly defined, as assisting Nature to regain that ascendancy by which she of her own accord will throw off what is offensive to her. The practitioner ought therefore to strengthen her in every possible way; and we have the latest discoveries of science as a guarantee that the present (the packing or wet-sheet process) method of carrying out the cure effectuates this end more completely than any other; what therefore is opposed to that, is so much drawn from the strength which it is the object to promote, and inasmuch as sweating, however it may tend to alleviate, undoubtedly weakens, it is a counteracting agency.

"Priessnitz is reaping the benefit of twenty years' experience. He follows still as he always followed (as far as it was possible for him to read and understand) the mysteries of his great mistress, Nature. Chance, I imagine, has in no way guided his choice; it may have assisted him in interpreting some of the revelations of this great spirit, but he has always had the same unerring basis on which to establish his system. Through imperfect light he may have sweated for a time, but the still small voice of truth has never ceased to whisper in his ear, and it is highly conducive to his honour that he should now have the courage to say that in this point he erred. He does this at the risk of reputation and fortune; he subjects himself to the abuse of high and low; but he acts up to his conviction, which is that the packing sheet, if to be persevered in, is better than the sweating process."

Though, however, the sweating process is not now so general, it is not entirely abandoned. A lady, a friend of mine, had a cold—she was ordered to sweat lightly twice a day, for two or three days. A gentleman had a swelling in his mouth; he was ordered the same. Others are ordered to sweat once or twice a-week, but the greater part of Priessnitz' patients never sweat at all.

Priessnitz guards people against the use of hot-air and vapour baths; they weaken and relax the skin. The difference between bringing a great amount of heat to act upon the surface, and causing the body to develop its own heat, must be obvious to every one.

XIV.—Sweating Process.

This process is precisely the same as that which has been already described, with the omission of the wet sheet. To produce perspiration, the body is enveloped in dry blankets. This tedious process in moderately strong people is seldom effected in less than three hours.

In the wet sheet, *no* water is given—but in the blankets, as soon as perspiration appears, it should be administered in small quantities; for this purpose a tea-pot is desirable.

In the Sweating process it is necessary to place a urinal in the bed of the patient. On proceeding to the bath after either of the operations, the attendant must take especial care to keep the body well covered, or his patient may take cold. On throwing off the covering, let the body be wetted all over instantly. This is an infallible precaution.

When there is a difficulty in procuring a bath, the dripping sheet full of water is used. If the first sheet does not cool, it must be repeated.

XV.—The Rubbing Sheet, or Abreibung.

This, by some, is called "the dripping sheet"; by others, "the wrung out" or "rubbing sheet." The term "rubbing" is used, because when the sheet is thrown on the body, great rubbing is used outside of it. It is a quick and simple mode of taking a general ablution; and, when frequently repeated, proves most effectual in restoring or increasing the circulation.

The value of friction to the human body is too well known to require observation. Hair gloves, hard brushes, or coarse towels cause a glow and an elastic feeling, though if long persevered in, they irritate and weaken the skin.

For the daily purposes of life, cold ablutions, and friction with dry cloths are sufficient; but to rouse the dormant energies, to give vitality to the system or combat illness, something more powerful is required.

The rubbing-sheet is a small sheet, soaked in cold water, and afterwards wrung out. This the attendant throws over the patient naked, who, standing up, receives it over his head and shoulders. When thus completely enveloped, the attendant rubs (outside the sheet) the back, loins, legs, and feet of the patient, whilst he himself rubs his abdomen and chest. The operation lasts about three minutes; the wet sheet is then replaced by a dry one, and friction again renewed until the body becomes quite dry; after which, if one rubbing-sheet only is prescribed, a waist-bandage is put on, a glass of water drank, and the invalid proceeds to take the air. If two or three rubbing sheets are prescribed, after the first operation as just described is over, the patient walks about the room in the dry sheet, with no other covering, for four or five minutes, occasionally approaching the window, which should be opened, throwing open the slight covering, in order to expose his skin to the air. The second and third rubbing-sheets are applied as the first.

Rubbing-sheets being used to effect several objects, are accordingly well wrung out, or not much wrung out, or scarcely wrung out at all. The first are used where there is a great want of vital energy, slow and languid circulation; the second is the ordinary mode of using the rubbing-sheet; the third is adopted where parties have lain in the packing-sheet or blankets and have no bath to cool them afterwards. Where there is a superabundance of heat, the rubbings are repeated perfectly wet, until the body is cooled.

The Rubbing Sheet is one of the safest and most efficacious appliances in the Water-cure. Every human body has in it 100½ degrees of heat; this is not diminished by the rubbing; by extracting we increase. Whenever persons are unwell, no matter the cause (except there may be eruptions on the body), a Rubbing Sheet is advisable. Where patients have been too exhausted to endure any other treatment, these sheets will resuscitate them in an extraordinary way.

Priessnitz perceived that merely rubbing the body with a damp and afterwards with a dry cloth was beneficial; but he found that whilst one part was under the operation, the other was exposed to catching cold; this gave him the idea of the Rubbing-Sheet, with which the whole body is covered at once.

As a general rule it is safe to begin the treatment of any illness with these sheets; they refresh the invalid, often ward off the complaint or develop the malady. In the cold stage of intermittent fever these rubbings down are persevered in until heat is produced; when the hot stage ensues, recourse is had to packing sheets, tepid baths, etc.

Where there is an excess of caloric, and fever is not declared, rubbing-sheets have a cooling effect, and often put an end to the illness at once. Where there is a want of caloric, as in ague, the Rubbing Sheets cause a determination of heat from the interior to the surface, in the same way that friction, or striking, brings heat out of matter. This may be elucidated by rubbing any part of the body with snow—re-action instantly ensues.

After great fatigue or a chill, or where persons have reason to think they have caught cold, two or three of these rubbings-down have an extraordinarily restorative effect.

They may be used by old or young, strong or weak, with perfect impunity.

In lumbago or rheumatism, or where it is necessary to rouse the vital energies, rubbing-sheets, four consecutively repeated, four times a-day, are frequently prescribed. A friend of mine, after getting wet whilst hunting, sat in his wet clothes, caught cold, and died. I am fully persuaded, if he had applied the Rubbing-sheets on getting home, the fatal result would have been avoided.

In some cases where a patient exhibits great weakness, languid circulation, and doubtful reaction, the sheet is wetted in tepid water, and sometimes the body is subjected to the action of cold by degrees, instead of being covered up at once, as is the case with the dripping sheet. There are invalids who cannot suffer anything cold to touch certain parts of their bodies; in such cases the tender part may be covered with a dry cloth, whilst the dripping sheet is applied, and the sensitive portion approached by degrees.

XVI.—The Douche Bath.

The douche, of all means employed, is the most powerful in stirring up, and removing humours from the position they may have occupied for years. What is understood by a "douche," is a spring of water, conveyed by pipes through the tops of small huts, from whence it falls in a stream about the thickness of one's wrist.

At Gräfenberg, there are six douches in the forest, with the falls of twenty feet, eighteen feet, and fifteen feet, respectively: the douches for women have a fall of only twelve feet, but no difference is made in the dimensions of the stream.

Patients are generally some time under the treatment before being permitted to take the douche. The douche is a most powerful stimulant.

As the sun by repulsion, brings heat out of matter, so the douche, by repelling, brings heat out of the body, and from the interior to the surface. It sets up a powerful action in the system, and is an active and useful agent for the cure of old-standing complaints. The douche should only be used in conjunction with other treatment.

The douche is never had recourse to in acute attacks; it is useful principally in chronic diseases. By its agency the body is hardened, and caused to develop its own force; it strengthens the skin, determines morbific matters to the surface by the pores, and exercises a powerful action upon the muscles and nervous system, by the action it provokes. In arthritic cases and rheumatism, the relief thus afforded is marvellous. It is so powerful a stimulant, that persons are frequently known, on coming out of the douche, to declare that they feel as much elation and buoyancy of spirits, as if they had been drinking freely of champagne.

A douche should be at some distance from the abode of the patient, because the necessary walk to it produces a glow of heat, and renders the body in a better state to produce re-action: no person should douche if cold or chilly.

The afflicted parts should be most exposed to the action of the douche, though it must be received successively upon all parts of the frame, except the head and face, unless otherwise prescribed. It should be avoided on the abdomen and chest when the latter is weak.

The douche ought to be discontinued when it produces feverish symptoms, and commenced again when they cease. The duration of it, in a general way, varies from two to five minutes, but is extended as the case may require, from fifteen minutes to half an hour; the latter being ordered in very especial cases.

An attendant waiting in the anti-chamber, throws a dry sheet on the patient on his coming out from the douche, rubs him dry, and puts on the waist bandage.

The time allotted for douching is two hours after breakfast, or dinner, but this rule is not without an exception; some patients, after their morning treatment, walk an hour, and then proceed to the Douche before breaking their fast.

Patients ought to be most particular in observing their doctor's orders in the use of the douche.

XVII.—The Shower Baths.

These baths so much recommended by the faculty are not used at Gräfenberg. Many persons in the habit of using them complain of giddiness and head-ache. This arises from the re-action upwards, which naturally results from their application. As an ablution, a bath, or washing with wet towels is preferable.

Mr. Priessnitz objects to the use of them, as parties take them without previous preparation, or other adjuncts. Falling on the head, they frequently cause congestion in that region.

XVIII.—The Sitz or Sitting Bath.

By this is to be understood a hip bath: that used at Gräfenberg is a small flat tub about seventeen inches in diameter and twelve or thirteen inches deep; a common washing tub placed against the wall will answer the purpose. The water in this bath is seldom more than four to six inches deep, in which the patient sits with his feet resting on the ground. No rule can be laid down for the duration of this bath, as it is ordered from ten minutes to an hour, and longer, depending upon the effect it is intended to produce. It is sometimes prescribed three or four times a day.

The sitting bath is of so much importance that where not prescribed the case is considered an exception to the ordinary rule of treatment. The sitting-bath cools and strengthens the viscera of the body, and by revulsion or derivation, draws the humours from the head, chest, and abdomen; relieves pain in the gums or face, and dissipates flatulency and cholic; and is of the utmost value to those who lead sedentary lives.

The object of using so little water in this bath, the foot and a half bath, is, that reaction may be the sooner effected. The water is only changed in peculiar cases. The abdomen should be well rubbed whilst taking the bath, and exercise taken immediately after it, to bring on a reaction. Where there is any tendency of heat or blood to the head, a wet bandage in the shape of a turban should be put on the head immediately before sitting in the bath, and continued the whole time. In commencing the hydropathic treatment, or where the patient is low spirited or unwell, or in cases where reaction is slow, a tepid sitting bath of 62 deg. to 64 deg. is usually prescribed. If a patient takes this bath immediately after the rubbing-sheet, or the room in which he takes it is cold, he should be covered with a cloak or dry blanket. Sitting baths must not be taken just before going to bed, excepting under peculiar circumstances.

In a case of asthma when the patient could hardly breathe, a tepid sitting bath relieved him effectually in fifteen minutes. In all cases of accidents to the head, evil consequences are averted by repeated sitting baths. Headaches are also generally relieved by these baths, which shows to demonstration that the theory of cold water when applied to the extremities driving the blood to the head, is completely devoid of foundation.

XIX.—Eye Bath.

As a preservative to the eyes, they should be kept open in a basin of water for two or three minutes every morning, or oftener. Glasses may also be used of the form of the eye, with water in them. For weak eyes, they are applied two or three times a day for five minutes each time. Where great inflammation exists, water should be thrown with the hand into the eyes several times a day.

XX.—Head Bath.

This bath can be taken in a common baking-dish, or any shallow vessel that can be kept flat on the ground. To take this bath, place a rug or blanket on the ground, and at the end of it, the vessel, containing water about two inches deep. The patient should extend himself on the rug so that his head may reach the dish or bason; then place the back of the head in the water, and keep it there three or four minutes; then each side of the head for the same time, and finish the operation by again subjecting the back of the head to the bath for two minutes. This process relieves headache. In cases of brain fever, and other diseases which cause great heat or pain in the head, these baths are frequently resorted to whilst the patient is in bed,—the back part of the head of the patient being placed in water, which is renewed when hot. In inflammation of the eyes, deafness, or loss of smell and taste, these baths are of great utility.

XXI.—Finger and Elbow Baths.

The wounded finger is placed in a glass of water; and there are cases where a glass is affixed by a string to the wrist, and the patient keeps the finger constantly in the bath. The elbow bath is used whenever the hand is wounded: it draws off the heat, and lowers the inflammation.

XXII.—Leg Bath.

The thighs and legs, when afflicted with ulcers, ringworms, etc., ought to be put into a bath, so as to cover the parts afflicted, for an hour or longer. This bath acts as a stimulant.

Other members of the body may likewise be subjected to baths; but their necessity must, be determined by circumstances.

XXIII.—Foot Bath.

This bath acts derivatively, and is employed as a counteracting agent against pains of the head, inflammation in the face, congestion to the upper regions of the body, fainting fits, bleeding of the nose, or spitting of blood.

Priessnitz prescribes cold foot-baths to effect the same object that the faculty endeavour to promote by warm ones.

The difference between a cold foot-bath and a warm one is, that after the cold one, a warm glow succeeds and remains; whilst cold feet are the necessary consequence of a warm bath. After the feet have been in cold water for some time, the water becomes tepid from the heat extracted. If the feet are put into hot water, heat, instead of being eliminated from the system, is brought to it—the very opposite to what is intended.

Sometimes, water at a temperature of 62 degrees is prescribed.

Cold foot-baths are accused of driving the blood to the head, for which notion there is not the slightest foundation, as the very opposite effect always attends their application. In the case of bleeding at the nose, I have seen them used several times; two cases, in fact, are worthy of notice:—A man was nearly exhausted from loss of blood from the nose; he put his feet into cold water, and the bleeding stopped in two minutes. A young lady, similarly attacked, put a key down the back and a wet towel upon the nape of the neck, without effect; her feet were put into cold water, and the bleeding ceased immediately. These two cases ought to satisfy the inquirer that cold foot-baths, far from causing congestion in the head, relieve the head.

Care must, however, be taken that the feet are warm when put into cold water, and exercise should be taken after the bath, in order to bring about re-action.

To prove that re-action always attends the use of these baths, when followed by proper exercise, we have but to observe our feet an hour or two after using one. After great fatigue a foot-bath is most refreshing. Mr. Priessnitz recommends the frequent use of these baths, as calculated to ward off complaints—many of which originate in the feet.

Friction and cold foot-baths are the best remedy for habitually cold feet.

Poor people who wear neither shoes or stockings, and whose feet are constantly exposed to a sort of foot-bath, avoid many complaints with which the rich are visited. It would be a misfortune to such people to be furnished with covering for the feet, as will be seen by two cases supplied me by friends on whom I can rely:—

An Irish gentleman, who removed a game-keeper from a low marshy estate to one high and dry, asked him one day how he liked the change. The man replied, "Not at all; he had never been well a day since he had been there, for there was not a drop of water to wet his feet."

A game-keeper, sent to prison to wait his trial for killing a man, being unwell, thought he would adopt his old habits as far as his confinement admitted of. He frequently immersed his feet in cold water, and kept them in motion. Soon after he began this, he recovered.

As a general foot-bath, the water should only come up to the instep; the feet and legs ought to be rubbed by an attendant, or one foot rubbed against the other the whole time. For cold feet ten minutes is sufficient, and the water need only cover the soles of the feet; but for other objects these baths are taken from fifteen minutes to half an hour, often much longer.

XXIV.—The Tepid, or Abgeschrecte Bath.

This bath is precisely the same as the half-bath, and applied in the same way; the only difference being the water, which in this bath is tepid; *i. e.* ordinarily 62 or 63 deg. of Fahrenheit, sometimes as high as 76 deg. In ordinary cases eight or ten minutes are sufficient, though in gout I have known it continued for hours. Great friction, except in eruptive cases, is applied the whole time.

The temperature during the use of this bath must be gradually diminished by the addition of cold water. After rubbing the body for a short time, the attendant throws a can of cold water on the head and shoulders and then renews the friction, a process repeated until inflammation and pain has subsided. If the patient feels weak or tired under the operation, he is allowed to come out for a few minutes and then begin again. It is customary with Priessnitz to put all new-comers into a tepid bath for one or two minutes, then into the cold plunge bath and back to the tepid. By these means he judges of their powers of re-action, and prescribes accordingly.

Tepid baths are always used in eruptive cases. All practitioners would do well to begin with these baths and proceed by degrees to colder ones. Every day's experience teaches Priessnitz the value of tepid baths.

Whenever these baths are ordered—for instance for fifteen minutes—instead of taking the whole at once, the dose is administered *à trois reprises*. After the first five minutes, the patient gets out of the bath and walks about the room, covered with a dry sheet, until he gains a little life and activity in the joints, which will be effected in two or three minutes. He then returns to the bath, and after the next five minutes the same process is repeated. After the third process, the patient is dried and walks about the room in the dry sheet for a short time, by way of taking an air bath. This is an important modification in the use of this bath. When patients are feeble and not able to support a bath so long as is often necessary to remove the attack, of whatever nature it may be, by dividing it in the way described, nature recovers herself a little during each rest, and the sufferer is thus enabled to take the whole; whereas, without any such pauses, the demand made on his strength might be too great. With children this mode of treatment is particularly observed.

XXV.—Bandages, or Umschlags.

Bandages fulfil two objects diametrically opposed to each other, viz., to calm and to stimulate. One object is effected by leaving a good deal of water in the bandage, not covering it with a dry one, and changing it as soon as hot. The other by wringing the bandage well out, covering it with a dry one and only changing it when dry.

1st. The more heat there is in the intestines the quicker the body bandages act.

2nd. Outward cold applications cause a fresh generation of heat.

3rd. By keeping the skin moist, these bandages cause the exudation of peccant humours and eliminate the excess of caloric.

4th. They equalise the temperature of the intestines, and keep up a healthy action in them.

5th. Wherever there is inflammation, their application and renewal lowers the temperature, and their moisture causes the healing of sores or wounds.

Those most in use, may be termed heating bandages. That for the waist, is worn day and night. It is 8½ feet long; eight or nine inches wide, with a double tape at the end to tie it with. To be put on with facility, it ought to be rolled up like a surgeon's bandage, beginning at the tape end. Then as much should be wetted and wrung out as will go once round the body, which the remaining part will cover. The chest bandages are made of coarse linen, *doubled*, in the shape of a breast-plate, to fit the chest and the throat, tied with three pair of tapes, one round the neck, under the arms, and round the waist. There must be two breast-plates, one to button into the other: the smaller to be wetted, the larger to be dry.

In the water-cure the waist bandage is changed in the morning, at noon, in the afternoon, and on going to bed.

A clammy heat almost immediately succeeds the application of this bandage: a sensation which one soon becomes accustomed to. Large or small bandages of this nature are applied in an infinity of cases. Those afflicted with complaints of the throat or chest, wear the chest bandage at night. Bandages are also applied to the feet and legs as derivatives; and to all wounds, bruises, diseased parts, or wherever pain is felt.

The humid heat of these bandages has a stimulating and absorbent property; they relieve the body of superfluous heat, and extract vitiated matters from the parts to which they are applied, as is frequently seen by the water in which they are washed. Moreover, they regulate the bowels, kidneys, &c.

Mercury is constantly drawn from the pores in these bandages.—Prince Leichtenstein, who had rubbed a light green ointment into his leg twelve months previously to going to Gräfenberg, found that for a fortnight it came out of the flesh by means of these bandages. Some medical men are sceptical on this subject: to be convinced of the truth let such go to Gräfenberg, where they may have constant evidence of the fact.

These bandages assuage pain, and aid in curing—better than ointments and plaisters[sic]. It is in vain that we seek to cure malignant ulcers retained in the system by impure blood with ointments. At Gräfenberg this is effected by the general cure, in which these bandages occupy so prominent a part.

These bandages are used by every patient, and must be renewed after every application of the treatment. If not mentioned in any of the following cases, the omission is unintentional, and those for the waist and diseased parts must be applied notwithstanding.

To any one who has never been in a Water-cure establishment, the application of these bandages will doubtless appear fraught with danger; but so little is this the case, that they are applied to age and decrepitude, to infants as soon as born, and to persons of weak, nervous, and delicate constitutions.

So far from colds being produced by these bandages, when covered with dry ones, we find invalids almost entirely encased in them nightly for months together. Let any one in pain, or who has a sore throat, try them, and he will soon be a convert to our opinion.

In inflammation, congestion of the blood, head-aches, burns, scalds, and wounds, until inflammation subsides, bandages without dry ones over them are used.

For this purpose, linen several times doubled, is wetted in cold water and placed upon the parts affected, where it remains until hot, and then is renewed until the disease ceases for which it was applied.

Sometimes these bandages are changed every ten minutes. In cases of wounds or fractures, sitz-baths accompany these bandages, as together they keep down inflammation.

In inflammation and fever, and in all cases of sickness, discomfort, pain or cramps, a larger bandage than usual is required: this is a sheet folded up and applied from the arm-pits to the thighs, and changed frequently. This large bandage is frequently ordered at night to sleep in, instead of the smaller one.

A gentleman, greatly afflicted, was packed up at night in a wet sheet, with a blanket loosely bound round him, his arms and feet being left free. This afforded him relief from pain. Of course, care was taken that perspiration did not ensue. In the morning the patient took his usual treatment.

The following interesting fact, confirming the advantage of bandages, is related in Baron Larry's "Memoir of the Russian Campaign." "An officer underwent amputation of an arm, after which the surgeon lost sight of him for some time. Two years subsequently, he met the officer in the saloons of Paris, who stated, that his wound had been completely cured by the constant application of cold wet bandages, which he wetted at the different rivulets he met with in his retreat, without any other application whatever."

In a Water-cure Establishment bandages are applied wherever pain or inconvenience is felt. Sometimes a patient has his legs, thighs, loins, and perhaps an arm or his head encased in them at one time, and so sleeps without any precautions as to increasing the amount of his covering.

A well-known English Gentleman caught leprosy in the East. Whilst under treatment at Gräfenberg, he slept in a pair of wet pantaloons, and a wet waistcoat covered with dry ones every night. The dry covering soon became wet, as did the blanket, when the patient felt chilly and uncomfortable, yet no cold resulted. The blanket which was used as a covering attracted the humidity. Priessnitz ordered a second blanket to be put over the first, which absorbed the damp from the first. After a couple of hours this was taken off and the under blanket was found dry: thus the patient was relieved of his discomfort.

A Gentleman afflicted with Lumbago was advised to bathe in the Serpentine in winter. After having done so, he dipped his shirt in the water, wrung it out, and put it on, then buttoning up well and putting on a great-coat and a large neckcloth, he proceeded briskly to Hampstead and back; this produced great heat, and cured the lumbago. These circumstances lead to the conviction that dangers attending the application of wet linen to our bodies, are less real than is represented. Thus, the airing of linen before a fire previous to wearing it, is of no advantage; the slight damp in it, on the contrary, excites the skin, and is more beneficial than otherwise.

One thing the reader's attention must be called to as an incontrovertible fact. No person ever caught a cold or suffered inconvenience from the application of wet sheets or bandages in the Water-cure.

XXVI.—Diet.

"It is not the plenty of meat," says Dr. Scott, "that nourishes, but a good digestion; neither is it the abundance of wealth that makes us happy, but the discreet using of it."

Whilst under treatment, patients partake of three meals, breakfast, dinner, and supper. The breakfast and supper consist of bread, butter, milk and fruit. Dinner ought to consist of plain food, that is to say, roast and boiled meat, poultry and vegetables, puddings and fruits; fish and soup are not recommended.

Priessnitz is not an advocate for what is considered highly nourishing food; he contends that quantity is more essential than quality. The act of feeding causes the stomach, like other members of the body, to perform its office.

A written case was presented to him of a person treating himself. Priessnitz approved of what was doing, until he came to where it was stated the patient ate roast beef and mutton daily—through this he struck his pen. This opinion of Priessnitz's seems confirmed by Dr. Beaumont of the United States, who made some useful experiments upon a young man named —— Martin, who was desperately, though not mortally, wounded, by the discharge of a gun, the contents of which entered the chest, and passed through the integuments of the stomach, so that the whole process of digestion was laid open to observation. The most important inferences arrived at by the doctor, from his observations, were—

1st.—*That all stimulating condiments are injurious to the healthy stomach.*

2ndly.—*That the use of ardent spirits if preserved in, produces disease in the stomach.*

3rdly.—*That bulk as well as nutriment is necessary to the articles of diet.*

4thly.—*That the digestibility of aliment does not depend upon the quantity of nutritient principles it contains.*

Dr. Beaumont further adds, "Here we have incontestable proof, that disease of the stomach was induced, and going on from bad to worse, in consequence of indulgence in ardent spirits, *although no prominent symptom made its appearance*, and —— Martin was, in his general habits, a healthy and sober man."

I put the following questions to Mr. Priessnitz:—"Is it requisite to eat meat every day?" "Yes, whilst under the treatment, because of the waste which the operations and consequent exertions occasion." "In cases of obstinate constipation, animal food must be partaken of sparingly?" "When not under Hydropathic treatment, meat should not be indulged in every day, except where parties are subjected to great exertion or hard labour, and even then it is better to avoid it occasionally. In fact, people would be more healthy if they only eat meat on alternate days, and if all their food were cold instead of hot."

From the habitual use of hot aliments the lining coat of the throat and stomach becomes distended and weak—hence bronchitis and weak digestion.

To the question as to drinking water. Priessnitz said, "Drink plentifully at every meal, finish by a tumbler or two, and don't fail drinking five or six glasses daily."

Experience which is better than a thousand theories, proves that after partaking of indigestible food, or eating too much, a few glasses of water relieve the stomach. One is at a loss to conceive why people should avoid drinking water at their meals, since none suffer from its use, and Nature seems to require it. Those who feel indisposed, by abstaining from food altogether for a day and drinking water, may frequently avoid a serious illness.

Butter is fat food and bad for delicate digestions. The leaner the food the better, to restore tone to the stomach and bowels. To people of strong digestions this does not apply.

If we look around us, we find that three-fourths of the human family live and labour, and digest, without tasting animal food; that the remaining fourth, who indulge in it, do more homage to Apothecaries' Hall than all the rest. But it is argued, much depends upon climate: then how shall we reconcile the rice of the East, the potato of Ireland, the oatmeal of Scotland, and the rye-bread of Poland? We can easily understand people in hot countries living upon rice, maccaroni[sic], etc.; but if what we understand by the term, nutritious food, is absolutely indispensable, how reconcile ourselves to the potato as the only food for the largest portion of the inhabitants of Ireland? Rye, which is the staff of life to the Poles, is a grain next in degree to wheat; then follow barley and oats. Potatoes are the very worst and lowest description of food. Rye-bread is as manna sent from heaven, in comparison with oatmeal, the chief food of the highlands of Scotland; yet we see strong healthy people in Ireland and Scotland, living solely upon these to a fine old age, without the assistance of the Pharmacopœia.

Does not this prove Mr. Priessnitz is right, when he says quantity is more essential than quality?

The great mass of mankind live on vegetable diet, which comprehends all the products of the earth. An author tells us, "Recent discoveries have shewn that vegetables contain the same elements as flesh: the same gluten, albumen, fibrin, and oily matters that exist in a beefsteak, are also found in our esculent vegetables."

Experience proves that vegetable diet is lighter and less liable to bring on disease, than one in which animal food largely prevails.

From an early period the philosophers of Greece,—from amongst whom we may cite Zeno, Plutarch, Porphyrus, and Plautinus,—advocated and practised an exclusively vegetable diet. The Pythagorean sages inculcated the same: hence the prevalence of rice diet over the vast and densely-peopled regions of Asia. Mahomet is said to have lived upon dates and water. It is related that the philanthropists, Swedenborg and Howard, were vegetarians; that Newton, Descartes, Haller, Hufeland, Byron, Shelley, and a host of other men of genius, were advocates of a vegetable diet. The continued use of meat produces scurvy, liver disease, rheumatism, gout, piles, etc.

Lamartine is a vegetarian.

On the score of economy, it is ascertained that the same plot of ground which would provide animal food for one man, would feed seventeen on vegetables.

For sick and delicate people, nutritious food should give way to coarser fare when under treatment. Priessnitz says he lost a colonel in the army, entirely from his indulgence in niceties and nourishing food; he could not be induced to confine himself to plain coarse fare: his digestion, in consequence, was always impaired.

Salt is injurious when acid humours or sores affect the body.

All spices, such as pepper, cloves, cinnamon, and mustard, are to be avoided, on account of their stimulating properties: nature gave these stimulants to the Indians, because their burning sky, by enervating the body, rendered them necessary.

In our climate the air is more compressed, and contains a larger amount of oxygen, which predisposes to inflammatory diseases. "Use," says Priessnitz, "the seasonings nature has given us, and leave to foreigners theirs: nature has provided for man's wants; our eatables ought, on that account, to agree with us the better."

Good household or brown bread is considered better than white bread.

Beer, wine, and alcohols of all kinds, are interdicted, as not assimilating with the food. It is a mistake to suppose that such things assist digestion: they have a totally opposite effect. Every museum of natural history exhibits substances preserved in wine, spirits of wine, or spirits, which would be dissolved in water.

A question arises, if, after having undergone the Water-cure, it is requisite to pursue any particular regimen? To this it may be answered, that those who continue a life of temperance stand a better chance of enjoying health and happiness than those who do not; but abstemiousness does not follow the Water-cure as a matter of course, any more than it does medical treatment. It is, however, necessary to abstain from intemperance for a short time after leaving off the treatment, or serious consequences may ensue.

To those who have passed the meridian of life, whose circulation is languid, who have been accustomed to stimulants, Mr. Priessnitz recommends the occasional use of light wines; and in speaking of wine as an alterative, he admitted that there could be no rule without an exception.

Tea and coffee attack the nerves. In my travels through Ireland, I was shocked at the ravages made upon the weaker sex by tea, the abuse of which has become a besetting sin. Give two or three cups of strong tea to one unaccustomed to it, and its effects will be evident upon the nervous system: in most cases it will deprive the recipient of sleep. I have known a strong man who, to cure headache, drank three or four cups of strong black tea, who, a few hours afterwards, trembled from head to foot. The same often attends the drinking of coffee. Dr. Sir Charles Scudamore, in his work on Hydropathy, states that Liebig, the best living chemical authority, said that coffee impeded the digestion of food for one or two hours, its carbonaceous principle requiring oxygen; and that he looked upon green tea as a poison. Tea and coffee-drinkers declare that neither affect them, and refer to persons who have drank both during a long life, and are, notwithstanding, in health. There are exceptions. The Bacchanalian, in like manner, justifies his revels, and the Turk his opium—but *"mark the end!"*

Stomachs weakened by the continued use of stimulants revolt at milk, which is the only food of most animals when young, and, as such, contains a large amount of nutriment, which is not the case with tea or coffee. I know a lady, the wife of one of Napoleon's marshals, who, for some complaint, was prescribed a milk diet. During a period of twenty years she has not taken an ounce of anything in the shape of food, having confined herself entirely to milk. Her health has been invariably good, and, though no longer young, can endure an excursion on foot over the mountains of Switzerland better than any of my female acquaintances. Does not this speak volumes in favour of milk as a diet for children or adults?

At Gräfenberg, patients who cannot drink milk mix it with water until the stomach gains tone; others drink sour milk, and find it agree with them, when common milk would not: this is to be accounted for from the milk having already undergone the first process of fermentation, which process would otherwise have taken place in the stomach. Most new-comers to Gräfenberg have a strong prejudice against sour milk, which, after persevering in taking it for some time, generally ends in their liking it exceedingly. Sour milk, with sugar and strawberries, is delicious. Boiled milk, with bread broken in it, agrees with most people, and makes a nourishing meal. To those with whom milk alone does not agree, cocoa, with plenty of milk, is recommended as wholesome and economical.

It has been observed by an able writer, that some people think that to live well means only to eat, and, it might be added, to drink. To hear that a man can enjoy the pleasures of the table, who refrains from wine and beer, and whose only beverage is water, appears paradoxical. Some go so far as to say that they prefer death to purchasing life on such terms, forgetting that a temporary indulgence at the table for a couple of hours may render them uncomfortable for the remainder of the twenty-four, and that the exciting, overcharging, and thickening of the blood, renders them hypochondriacal and morose, and makes invalids of men who ought to be in the enjoyment of robust health. It is hardly to be expected that nature will deal mercifully with him who has for so many years sinned against her mandates: she will, doubtless, sooner or later reward the crimes of *lèse majesté* committed against her high prerogatives.

> "Nothing like the simple element dilutes
> The food, or gives the chyle so soon to flow."

The *bon-vivant*, from the excited state of his system, is not only more subject to complaints than persons who live temperately, but is more difficult of cure. When overtaken with pain and illness, notwithstanding his stoicism in declaring for a short life and a merry one, no one desires to be restored to health with greater earnestness, or manifests a more ardent clinging to life than himself.

Priessnitz's assumption that the indigenous products of the country wherein we reside being best calculated for the support of health, is borne out by Liebig, who says: "Even when we consume equal weights of food in cold and warm countries, infinite wisdom has so arranged that the articles of food of different climates are most *un*equal in the proportion of carbon they contain. The fruits on which the natives of the South prefer to feed, do not, in the fresh state, contain more than 12 per cent. of carbon; whilst the bacon and train oil used by the inhabitants of the Arctic regions, contain 66 to 80 per cent. of carbon."

Avoiding all excess, it is man's prerogative to elaborate and assimilate the most heterogeneous aliments, not being limited, like other animals, to any particular food; and it is certain that those who approach nearest to nature, who enjoy the benefit of pure air and lead an active life, do not require to observe any particular rules.

One thing, however, is admitted: the duration of life depends upon the simplicity of our wants. Most people eat too much, especially of animal food. No people talk so much of indigestion, dyspepsia, and constipation, as the English; it has been said that they take more pills and aperients, and pay more fees, than all the nations of the world together! What a distinction from savage life! The child of nature, whose only drink is water, can, without inconvenience, go for days together without food, and then commit excesses that, if indulged in in civilised life, would produce fatal results.

It ought to be observed, that abstinence from wine and spices is compensated by the pleasure water-drinkers take in being enabled to partake *ad libitum*, of pastry, fruit, and other delicacies of the table, which wine-drinkers dare not indulge in.

XXVII.—Clothing, Air Baths, Wearing Stays, etc.

Mr. Priessnitz expects all his patients to leave off wearing flannel or cotton next to the body; he maintains that by keeping up too much heat, they weaken the skin, which then is less efficient in performing its offices, and in consequence people become delicate and diseased.

A patient coming out of the bath, on being prevented putting on his flannel waistcoat and drawers, said, "Tell Mr. Priessnitz, they and I having been intimately acquainted for twenty years, I hardly like parting with them so abruptly." His reply was, "They are false friends; in a short time your skin will regain the proper tone which they deprived it of, when you will be warmer without flannel than ever you were with it." Priessnitz does not preach one doctrine and practise another—he wears nothing under his linen. Some patients of a slow circulation, on commencing the treatment, are ordered to wear their flannel waistcoats over their linen for a few days: the want of it is not felt. It might naturally be supposed, that leaving off flannel of a sudden, especially in cold weather, would be attended with serious consequences; but this is never the case in the Water-cure. Invalids frequently arrive at Gräfenberg in the depth of winter, and after the bath, invariably leave off flannel. Of the number of cases that came under my observation, I never knew a single instance of a party catching cold. After the bath, the patient is expected to keep up a brisk walk for some time. In winter, it would be as well, after leaving off flannel, to clothe warmer than usual for a day or two.

Wearing flannel waistcoats in bed of a night is greatly debilitating. An almost universal prejudice exists in favour of flannel in cases of gout and rheumatism; hence the question arises, "Does it prevent or cure those complaints?" Certainly not; for where do you see their victims without flannel? Experience proves, that it neither protects the wearer from disease, nor allays pain.

Nightcaps destroy the hair, cause its premature decay, and have an injurious tendency to those troubled with congestion in the head, head-aches, etc.; such people cannot have their bedrooms too cold. There is much sense in the old adage—"Keep the head cold, and the feet warm." Previously to sleeping without a nightcap, and washing my head every morning with cold water, I was constantly tormented with cold in the head, from which I am now perfectly free. Perhaps, in some measure, I am indebted to my last visit to Gräfenberg for this happy change, having passed a whole winter there without wearing either hat or neck-cloth, or making any change from my summer clothing, although the thermometer was frequently 12° to 14° Reaumur below zero.

The constant use of oils and pomatums to the hair, unless the head is often washed, closes the pores, and is prejudicial.

With respect to the clothing, Priessnitz advises "when in an open carriage, or sitting still, the body should be well clothed; when in exercise, as lightly covered as possible."

One half the cases of consumption in females may be traced to the wearing of stays, and lacing them too tight. All artists agree, that stays in growing people destroy, rather than improve, the figure. Bound up in whalebone, they lose that graceful undulation of the back which is so pleasing. Every one who has seen the Venus de Medicis, Canova's Venus, or any other faithful copy of nature, must consider a very small waist a defect.

Stays, at best, are unwholesome, as they keep up an unnatural heat about the body; and when laced too tight, are sure to be attended with serious consequences. I have known several young ladies, whose teeth were destroyed, whose breaths were intolerable, and who were consigned to a premature grave, entirely from tight lacing. To have health, the greatest of all blessings, the complicated machinery inside our bodies must have room for action (the intestinal canal, for instance, is half as thick as a man's arm, and sixty or seventy yards long); contract this space, you contract the vessels, and irregularity of the functions ensues. This is an offence against nature, which sooner or later she will repay with misery and pain.

Dr. Abernethy advised air baths, that is, the habit of exposing the body naked to the air, which may be done with impunity after the cold bath, but not otherwise. In winter, instead of increasing the amount of clothing, Priessnitz advises exercise; for, in proportion as the body is warmly clothed, and the air excluded, the less warmth is produced by the body itself; resistance to cold causes the body to bring forth its own energies and powers. There can be no doubt the feet are much warmer, and that it is much healthier, to go without stockings; it necessitates washing the feet oftener, which, if done in cold water, tends to bring warmth to them. The Turks owe much of their health to their habit of washing their feet. Before going to Gräfenberg, people destitute of shoes and stockings excited my pity; but since that time, my opinion is changed: let such persons be well fed, but for health keep their feet bare. The following extracts from Liebig support Priessnitz's opinion:—

"Our clothing is merely an equivalent for a certain amount of food. The more we are clothed, the less urgent becomes the appetite for food; because the loss of heat by cooling, and consequently the amount of heat to be supplied by the food, is diminished.

"If we were to go naked, like certain savage tribes; or if in hunting or fishing, we were exposed to the same degree of cold as the Samoyedes, we should be able with ease to consume ten pounds of flesh, and perhaps a dozen of tallow candles into the bargain, daily; as warm-clad travellers have related with astonishment of those people."

"The Englishman, in Jamaica, feels with regret the disappearance of his appetite, previously a source of frequently recurring enjoyment. And he succeeds by the use of cayenne pepper and the most powerful stimulants, in enabling himself to take as much food as he was accustomed to eat at home. But the whole of the carbon thus introduced into the system is not consumed; the temperature of the air is too high, and the oppressive heat does not allow him to increase the number of respirations by active exercise, and thus to proportion the waste to the amount of food taken; disease of some kind, therefore, ensues."

"The cooling of the body, by whatever cause it may be produced, increases the amount of food necessary, the mere exposure to the open air, in a carriage or on the deck of a ship, by increasing radiation and evaporation, increases the loss of heat and compels us to eat more than usual. The same is true of those who are accustomed to *drink large quantities of water*, which is given off at a temperature of the body 98°. It increases the appetite; and persons of weak constitution find it necessary, by continued exercise, to supply to the system the oxygen required to restore the heat abstracted by the cold water. Loud and long continued speaking, the crying of infants, and moist air, all exert a decided and appreciable influence on the amount of food which is taken."—LIEBIG.

"No isolated fact," says Dr. Johnson, "can contravene the law that the quantity of food is regulated by the number of respirations, by the temperature of the air, and by the amount of heat given off to the surrounding medium, as for instance by frequent bathing. Of course it is a matter of indifference whether that medium be cold air or cold water."

As a healthy naked body generates by heightened perspiration of the skin, the same warmth as is produced by one which is covered, by means of retaining the perspiration; so every one who is quite well, might by use become so hardened, that during the coldest season he might feel, when naked, as comfortable as any one covered with wool. The truth of this was verified by two English gentlemen, the winter I spent at Gräfenberg. One day in December, when the thermometer was at 6°, of Reaumur, below zero, they proceeded to a mountain, took off all their clothes, except their drawers, and proceeded to the top, where, though the wind was blowing strong at the time, they remained two hours. They stated that after they had walked briskly, or got up the steam for ten minutes, a glow of heat came on, which counteracting the cold, produced the most agreeable sensation. Neither of these gentlemen caught cold or suffered in any way from this experiment.

The Scotch Highlander with his naked legs, does not feel colder, surrounded by mountains of ice, than we do who are clothed. We prove this by our bare faces in the coldest winter.

As the skin performs the double function, of drawing nourishment from the air, and exhaling the phlogisticised air of the diseased matter and worn-out atoms of the body, it follows that the true art of curing, must be to endeavour to restore these two functions. Hydropathy causes the ejection of diseased matter and revives the activity of the skin.

Dr. Johnson observes, "Discomforts are the necessary whips and spurs which keep the living energies awake; whilst comforts operate upon us like opiates: since to acquire a 'comfort' is only to remove a discomfort; and to remove what keeps us awake, is the same thing as to administer what will send us to sleep. The indulgences, therefore, wherewith even young and healthy men indulge themselves; the 'comforts,' as they call them, of flannel, warm clothing, closed doors, carpeted rooms, soft beds, hot food, are infinitely worse than absurd; because the opposites of all these luxuries, so far from being injurious to health, are absolutely *necessary* to it. We actually kill ourselves with comforts."

XXVIII.—Drugs.

"Thus with our hellish drugs, Death's ceaseless fountains
In these bright vales, o'er these green mountains
    Worse than the very plague we raged.
I have myself to thousands poison given,
And hear their murderer praised as blest by heaven,
    Because with Nature strife he waged."

Göethe's Faust.

The influence of habit and custom is such, that it is difficult to arouse inquiry, when the result is calculated to derange the existing order of things. Mr. D'Israeli observes, "Could we conceive that man had never discovered the practice of washing his hands, but cleansed them as animals do their paws, he would for certain have ridiculed and protested against the inventor of soap, and as tardily, as in other matters, have adopted the invention."

All change, however beneficial, is attended with trouble; and we therefore adopt the motto, "Whatever is, is right." This very motto is the key to our method of cure—as it is to that of every other great moral truth. Yet, to quote the words of Rausse, "We do not take this in the sense of the philosophy of our days, or in that of the German philosopher, Hegel, for then we must consider falsehood and assassination to be good. Rather would we take these words in the sense in which they were first proclaimed by the philosophy of Geneva, in the sense in which the *first citizen* used them for the foundation of his truths; thus, that which is produced by nature is good; all inclinations, all impulses of men derived from nature, are good; and every mis-usage of nature is an outrage which she punishes with misery and pain. All the principles of the art of curing at Gräfenberg, attested as they are by thousands, are dictated by that instinct which nature has given to every human being as his inheritance."

But are not all the cures performed at Gräfenberg—all the doctrines of Hydropathy—opposed to science? It may be answered, Yes; nor can we shut our eyes to the fact, that nature refuses all respect for what we are pleased to denominate learning—nay, tramples upon what is often called science: particularly on that of medicine. By what delusions were mankind first persuaded to submit to the use of poisonous drugs! In the middle ages, water as a beverage, and as a cure for disease, fell into total disuse. In the time of the Crusades, the Arab doctors introduced the use of Oriental drugs, to which they attributed miraculous virtues; and during the period of astrology and alchemy, and when researches were being made for the philosopher's stone, almost every nation boasted of having found some panacea—some elixir vitæ: sometimes it was an oil or an herb; at others, a powder or mineral; until, in process of time, their accumulation formed the vaunted science of medicine. But, we would inquire, are the effects of these compounds such as to lead to the conclusion that they were recommended by nature? Have mankind become healthier since their introduction? Are those nations who have done most homage to this science, the strongest and soundest?

To think of eradicating disease with poisons, of which physic is generally composed, appears paradoxical. How is it possible to bring physic to bear upon the dispersed and deeply-hidden diseased matter? Even if this could be done, it is quite impossible, as every chemist knows, for the peccant matters and physic to dissolve each other into nothing.

Dr. Forbes, editor of the "British and Foreign Medical Review," supports this view of the case. He observes, "It is one of the most formidable difficulties with which the ordinary physician has to contend, that nearly all his remedies reach the point to which they are directed, through one channel. If the brain requires to be placed under the influence of a sedative or a stimulant, if the muscular system demands invigorating by tonics, if the functions of organic life need correction by alteratives, the physician has no means of attaining his object except by inundating the stomach and bowels with foreign and frequently pernicious substances. It being thus made the medical doorway to all parts of the system, and so compelled to admit every description of therapeutical appliances, the organ of digestion is contorted to a purpose for which it was never intended."

"The consequence," says Dr. Arbuthnot, "of such treatment with physic is, that to the old evil a new stimulus is added, weak or strong, according to the dose and quality: what is inflammable, stays in the blood, and afterwards affects the brain."

We may fairly ask, How can any of these consequences result from Hydropathy? The following lines of Horace Smith are not far from the truth:—

> "Physic! a freak of times and modes,
> Which yearly old mistakes explodes
>   For new ones still absurder.
> All slay,—their victims disappear,
> And only leaves the doctrine clear
>   That killing is no murder."

Are those who do most to aid the apothecaries, and who indulge in alcoholic drinks, healthier than others; or, are those who are in the habit of consulting doctors free from pain? No! they drag on a miserable existence. It might be asked, If certain herbs and minerals were alone intended for healing man's infirmities, how would the inhabitants of the temperate zone procure those that are indigenous to the tropics, and *vice versâ*? Instinct pleads in favour of the element that abounds wherever human beings ought to live; and innumerable instances might be adduced of the advantage which the use of water gives the savage over cultivated man.

From the most remote ages, water was known and resorted to as a curative agent by the unsophisticated children of nature. In the wilds of America, the savage is put into a close hut, built of stones, which hut is heated to produce intense perspiration on the invalid, in which state he is immersed in the river, near to which the hut is generally placed; and by Pallme's travels in Kordofan, we find that, in the very depths of Africa, fevers are cured by cold water. It appears our traveller lay several days in bed with burning fever, when, at length, his attendants lifted him out of bed, placed him with his back against the door, and poured a large volume of cold water on his head and body. After the shock he was put to bed, covered with sacks and sheepskins: this produced relief and sleep. A second application of this treatment effected a cure.

Some writers err in supposing mankind to have arrived at an age of decrepitude, from its not occurring to them that the deterioration of health arises from art, and not nature. If you wish to be convinced of this, leave civilised and go to savage life. There you will see the man of nature as young and strong as the first created; the generation cannot grow old, except by art, poison, or vice. Prescribe simple water, and it is rejected with scorn; but let any quack recommend his drugs, however poisonous, and they are swallowed regardless of results. It must have been the enemy of all good who first persuaded mankind that poison could produce health.

The evils that arise from pernicious drugs, which have swept away millions, and which will destroy the whole species if no reform takes place, originate in misunderstanding the first or acute attack, which is but an attempt of nature to heal. Men take acute attacks for disease, whilst *in reality they are the means by which the system is relieved of disease*. Bleeding, blistering, cupping, and drugging, subdue these efforts,—not by emancipating the system, but by so reducing it that it can no longer contend with its enemy. Men praised the unlucky discovery, and hence a host of deadly diseases took their origin, such as destructions and suppurations of the inner organs, dropsy, etc.: complaints which were hardly known in times of yore, and which, but for these causes, would never have reared their heads. However, as the lamentable consequences in some cases do not appear until years after the suppression of the acute conflict, no one thinks of attributing them to drugs. This drug-plague is the most dreadful malady mankind has to contend with; dug by themselves from the black abysses of the earth, it has been cherished as the effect of deep science for centuries; how frequently has the last shilling been offered up at its altar! Upon it as many millions have been spent as would pay off the National Debt: to the study of these dangerous errors, millions of men have applied the whole of their lives and their ability: backed by this so-called science, they contend against nature; but *how* does Nature punish those who wish to master her? Oh, great unspeakable Nature! how dreadfully beautiful art thou, in thy inexorable and destroying severity!

Mankind may still turn back, and regenerate health; but it is not sufficient for them to renounce physic: they must abandon wine, spirits, and poison, in every shape. For the curing of disease, we must not look into the grey mysteries of the future, but far behind us, on the green plain of Nature, and of the times which are past.

XXIX.—Assimilation.

The preservation of life requires not only that its consumption should be reduced, but its restoration rendered more easy. For this purpose two things are necessary, the perfect assimilation of that which is beneficial, the separation from that which is injurious. Life, as will be seen from the following definition, depends upon the identification, the assimilation, and the animalisation of external matter by the vital power, in its passage from the chemical to the organic world.

The power of assimilating other substances into itself is the fundamental principle of nature. This impulse and power is not only prevalent in all organic matter, but also in elemental bodies, that is to say, water, earth, and fire. The globe in the beginning was a rigid rock, upon which air and water effected their power of assimilation.

Assimilation is only possible by dissolving. For the purpose of assimilation, air and water dissolved the earth's crust; by the agency of those powers that surface originated which produces and nourishes all organic bodies. As these exist in the same world in which the elements continually exercise their power of dissolving and assimilating, it follows, that from the beginning there must have been developed in all organic elements the same power, as a protection to themselves.

Air dissolves water into vapours, in order to assimilate gases from it. Water extracts from air the oxygen gas.

Fire absorbs the oxygen of air, dissolves water into its two component parts, hydrogen and oxygen, and by converting the former to a flame, transforms water to fire; air absorbs many gases which fire releases from combustibles; air draws gases from the soil, the soil absorbs the oxygen of the air. In this way the elements are in a constant conflict, each endeavouring to dissolve the other, and to assimilate its matters with itself. Organic bodies draw oxygen from the air by the process of respiration, which is also the property of plants: these draw all assimilatory matter which the earth offers by their roots. The same process is performed by animals feeding on plants or herbs; whereas, on the contrary, fire resolves all organic matter into its original elements. This same process is carried out by water and air, with all organic beings, but as long as these are living they only get their evaporation, and after death their entirety. The earth exercises this power but conditionally and partially, viz. upon all animals that exist in it, and on all roots of plants; upon mankind the earth only exercises its power of assimilation after death. The proofs of this conflict of assimilation in organic matter itself are clear, one animal eats the other as well as plants; that is to say, it absorbs by the agency of the stomach so much of their substance as may be assimilated. Plants again convert parts of dead bodies and other plants (the manure) into their own substance.

Besides this power of assimilation, there exists in every being, element and organisation, the necessity of being exposed to foreign assimilation.

This is the fundamental principle of the true doctrine of healing. In support of this theory, we find that water, if withdrawn from the power of dissolution by the fresh air, stinks and putrefies. Air loses its oxygen and becomes mephitic, if it does not find water or plants with which it can enter into the conflict of dissolution and assimilation.

Animals and plants fall ill and die if their surface is so covered that neither air nor water can act upon them. If nourishment is withdrawn from any organic being, that is to say, if it is deprived of the opportunity of assimilating with external or foreign substances, death is caused by the want of a supply of healthy juices; if, on the contrary, this being is deprived of the influence or effect of this foreign power of dissolution, illness is the consequence, arising from the putridity of matter, from which putridity the system ought to have been released by the agency of foreign assimilation.

XXX.—THE CRISIS.

"Most blessed water! neither tongue can tell
    The blessedness thereof, nor heart can think,
Save only those to whom it hath been given
To taste of that divinest gift of heaven.

"I stoop'd and drank of that divinest well,
    Fresh from the Rock of Ages where it ran,
It had a heavenly quality to quell
    All pain: I rose a renovated man;
And would not now, when that relief was known
For worlds the needful suffering have forgone."

To those unaccustomed to the Water-cure treatment, the Crisis is looked upon as something beyond human endurance; but by those who understand the nature of it, its arrival is hailed with joy, as the forerunner of a favourable termination to their sufferings. A Crisis has a two-fold object, the restoration of the animal functions to the condition of health, and the cure of a disease. It is not therefore a necessary consequence of the treatment; since, if there be no disease, the body is free from vitiated matter, and no eruption can appear; but if noxious matters exist in the system, whatever temporary relief be obtained by drugs or ointment, no permanent beneficial effect can be produced until they are extracted. Otherwise, original health, that is, the same muscular power and elasticity of body proportionately dealt out to all animals, will never be obtained during the life of an individual. Nature, to effect the elimination of non-nutritious matter, may resort to measures imperceptible to the patient, such as evaporation caused by ablutions, by relaxation of the bowels, or other evacuatory means. Although for twelve months, whilst at Gräfenberg, I went through all the necessary processes, I never had any perceptible crisis, except a slight water-rash, and the same may be said of many friends of mine, who have passed through the treatment.

There is a critical period, if the treatment is persevered in: it is when Nature is about to resume her power over the disease, the latter having been attacked, and seeking to escape. It may be compared to a tiger which a man is tempting in his lair: for a time, it lies dormant, occasionally giving signs of existence, when suddenly the animal rouses, and a violent struggle ensues. The man however proves the strongest of the two. In all future attacks too, which are less vigorous, the tiger is defeated, until he finally quits his lair, and flies from his human conqueror. Thus at last are old diseases eradicated. In acute cases, the first rencontre often settles the affair.

Under the Water-cure it frequently happens that every evil and pain is increased in intensity from the fact of the strength being always progressing. The weak and debilitated feel little pain; feebleness has produced insensibility. As the vital force diminishes, in the same proportion are the symptoms less violent; but when strength and vigour are daily gaining ground, so do the symptoms become more vigorous and intense. Nature is in a state of revolution; and, by being reinstated in her rights, she has declared war with all foreign powers that ventured to invest her citadel, and trample upon her rights and laws during the period of her prostration.

An officer in the Prussian army, author of the most concise and best-written work on the Water-cure, told me that at Gräfenberg six years ago he was radically cured of a complication of diseases: that he had the so-called crisis; the first attack was painful and distressing in the extreme; rheumatism returned to each part where he had previously felt it; his foot, which some years before had been trodden upon by a horse, became exceedingly painful; his hands and feet swelled to double their ordinary size, and there was a discharge of an offensive nature from them. This lasted for about ten days. In the course of his cure he had two other attacks, each inferior in intensity to the preceding one. After the last, he found his hearing, of which he had been deprived two years, restored; he could walk as well as ever he did, a necessary pleasure of which rheumatism had deprived him; in fact, he left Gräfenberg a new man, and has ever since been perfectly well. This gentleman said that, whilst in a fortress, with his regiment, almost all the officers, except himself, suffered from influenza, whilst he escaped, from drinking cold water and taking several ablutions a day.

When a crisis is expected, Priessnitz increases the treatment, as he also does when it has made its appearance: instead of discouraging the crisis to proceed, he encourages it by all the means in his power. So that eruptions, boils, fever, diarrhœa, inflammation, or aught else brought out by the treatment, may be gradually reduced by it. In this stage of the Water-cure, no compromise can be made; the fight must be continued until the enemy quits the field.

A lady of my acquaintance, on the appearance of an eruption, gave up the treatment until it disappeared; the eruption took an inward direction and inflammation of the lungs was the consequence: the most vigorous measures were now resorted to by Priessnitz, or her life would, most probably, have paid the forfeit. Another lady was treating herself to great advantage. After some time, when some boils made their appearance, she became uneasy and low-spirited. Alarmed, she left off the cure; the boils receded, and a fever succeeded them, which, as she could not procure advice, ended in a painful illness. When hydropathy was first introduced into England, the death of a clergyman, who had been treated by it, caused a great sensation. This gentleman went to an establishment on the Rhine, where he staid two or three months: on his determining to leave, the doctor, who saw indications of a Crisis, advised him to stay. The patient disregarded this advice and proceeded home; when, as predicted, a number of boils appeared. Mistaking these friends for enemies, he sent for a medical man, who declared the boils to arise from poverty of the blood, administered something to cause them to retire, and advised him to drink wine and beer, and live freely. As might have been expected, the result was fatal.

Had this gentleman been subjected to the Packing-sheet followed by Tepid-bathing; and had the boils been constantly bandaged, his health would, doubtless, have been improved.

I have known patients, whose blood was in an unhealthy state, throw out boils for months; but who, from constantly applying bandages to them, suffered but little inconvenience.

At some of the establishments in Germany, when a crisis is indicated, it is the practice to recommend patients to diminish the treatment or quit it altogether, thus throwing away the golden opportunity of realising health. Whilst at others with a limited knowledge of the Hydropathic treatment, some practitioners resort to Allopathic or Homoæpathic means of mitigating nature's effort to escape her bonds. Let not such men be trusted: they know not what they do. When in Ireland, I treated a person of advanced age who had been confined to bed for twelve months. In two days he was able to walk out on crutches. After I left, a large boil came in his back: not understanding the matter he gave up the treatment. Instead of the boil being forced to a head, it retired, and he fell into his old state. Had this boil been encouraged to a large size, the patient would, after its bursting, have felt much relief.

It is a common practice, under medical treatment, to open a boil, and thus put an end to it—a quick method, no doubt, of affording relief; but the morbific matters that could have accumulated there, and been eliminated by it, remain in the system. Fevers again, under our medical treatment, are suppressed; whilst in the Water-cure, the morbific heat is extracted by the pores, and the whole system cooled through the medium of the mucous membrane or skin.

It is in a crisis, that the mind of the great Water-king is made manifest. Such is the unbounded confidence of patients in him, that most of them ardently desire to pass through this ordeal. It must be observed, that, though it is sometimes a painful period, the assuaging power of the bandages, the non-necessity of confinement or abstinence from the usual diet, and the perfect security every one feels as to the result, renders it endurable. It is at the same time equally true, and worthy the attention of any one about to undertake the cure, that during the revivifying process, weakness and lassitude are the pregnant attendants of the early part of it; and greatly disappointed would be that new aspirant to health who should fancy that all was *couleur de rose*. It is an old saying, and perhaps true, that all good things cost money or trouble; and the attainment of health, by the removal of long-standing complaints through the water-cure, is no exception to the rule. It is a delusion to suppose that inveterate diseases are to be cured by the water treatment, as by miracle, without suffering. Moral energy and firmness are necessary to go right through the ordeal. In such circumstances the patient must exert all his fortitude to adhere strictly to the instructions that are given to him.

XXXI.—Dropsy.

A frequent argument made use of against drinking water is, that it produces dropsy. Now, if this were true, it must be evident such a complaint ought not to exist amongst us—for whoever heard of an Englishman drinking too much water? On the contrary, the English nation is remarkable for an almost hydrophobic dislike to it.

The more the human body has been saturated with drugs, alcohols, and other foreign matters, the greater is the necessity for a free action of the pores and perspiration, because by these agents it seeks to relieve itself of diseased matter. When the skin is relaxed or incumbered by that oily exhalation which is constantly exuding from the pores, and too often suffered to remain on the surface, fluids collect beneath the skin and cause inflammation—this is called dropsy.

One of the greatest promoters of dropsy, as every medical man knows, is the lancet, by which the good blood is extracted and a watery fluid substituted. Strong poisons of whatever nature they may be, either mercury, blue pill, calomel, bark, iodine, or any other of the ten thousand drugs from which relief is sought, and for which alcohols or other stimulants are persevered in, tend to vitiate the juices, and produce gout, dropsy, and numberless complaints from which the habitual water-drinker is exempt.

No modern writer on dropsy attributes it to drinking water, nor, observes Dr. Johnson, is there anything in the physiology of the capillary system of vessels which can warrant such an opinion; on the contrary, *drinking largely of diluting liquids is always recommended as an important part* of the cure of dropsy. Dr. Gregory, author of the Theory and Practice of Medicine, states that "no diuretic medicines are likely to be of service, without very copious dilution;" and adds, "*there cannot be a greater error* than to imagine that dropsical accumulations may be lessened by withholding liquid."

From the returns of 1841, within the city of London and bills of mortality, amongst a people opposed to the use of cold water in any way, we find that from dropsy alone the deaths amounted to 584.

Is not this fact alone sufficient to carry conviction to our minds, that dropsy is not the effect of water drinking? It may be safely affirmed that those who never take physic and who adhere to a water diet, will never be attacked with dropsy.

This complaint, except when of long standing, or under very extraordinary circumstances, is generally curable.

XXXII.—Smoking.

"Though smoking is decidedly prejudicial to health, it is not so bad as drinking to excess."

"Smoking irritates the nerves and promotes the secretion of saliva, which is withdrawn from digestion."[5]

"By blunting the nerves, a man, as in drinking, may stand a great deal of smoking without being visibly affected by it."

"A person who, previously to undergoing the water-cure, could drink a gallon of fermented liquor, may, after it, be affected by a single glass—from the fact of his nerves having recovered their sensibility."

"Persons who previously to the treatment were great smokers, are frequently rendered ill by very little smoking after it."

"The nerves are strong and vigorous in proportion to their sensibility and freshness.—He who goes through a thorough water-cure treatment, gains a great moral as well as physical command over himself."

"It is generally the weak and debilitated who are the most sensual and debauched."

"The sound man has purer tastes, independent of his greater self-command."

"We find amongst the children of nature, amongst simple peasants who have had but little contact with civilisation, the purest virtue and truest feelings of honor."—PRIESSNITZ.

OBSERVATIONS.—Persons who consider themselves in health, will derive advantage by six weeks' or two months' treatment at Gräfenberg, and will learn how to apply it to themselves or families.

Parents will there acquire the habit of using cold water, be prepared to ward off disease from themselves, and learn, by simple means, how to preserve the health of their children.

Officers in the army, who have an insight into hydropathy, will have nothing to fear from epidemics; they will find that fevers and inflammations are diseases which form the easiest part of Mr. Priessnitz' practice.

The water at Gräfenberg has no advantage over that which we find everywhere, except that it is peculiarly cold and fresh. In the general purposes of the cure, water should be soft, that is to say, it must possess the quality of dissolving, and for this reason it must be cold, and divested of all mineral properties; for to prove its fitness, linen cloth washed in it must become white, and vegetables dressed in it tender. Trout living in water does not prove its softness, but frogs do; the softest of all waters is the rain. Hard water makes the skin rough, but soft water, on the contrary, renders it smooth. When water, with the slightest acidity in it, has been suffered to remain in leaden pipes, pumps or cisterns for any length of time, it absorbs the dangerous qualities of the lead; and this has been known to produce serious consequences. It is necessary, therefore, that water should be drawn off before any is drunk.

Those who wish to begin ablutions in winter, should do so in a warm room, and as a beginning, instead of washing, they may wet a towel, and with it be well rubbed all over twice a day, or use the rubbing-sheet. The morning immediately on getting out of bed, is the best time for the first ablution; the other should be undertaken two or three hours after eating, *never* on a full stomach, nor immediately after making any great exertion. The rubbing should be continued from three to five minutes.

It is conceived that one ablution a-day, and the drinking of cold water, will enable those who are in health, and in the enjoyment of life, to continue in that state. After any excess, instead of resorting to drugs, the rubbing sheet should be resorted to, and an increase in cold water as a beverage. The same means may be resorted to by persons who have any reason to suppose that they have caught cold.

In answer to the question, whether there is not some risk of catching cold whilst washing, we answer, "Not the least." There is no better way of guarding against colds, or of hardening the skin, to contend with atmospheric changes. But in cold weather it is as well that all the body should be wetted simultaneously. Even in cold weather the temperature of the room to which the body is exposed, is higher or warmer than the water used, which cannot, in consequence, produce a cold. The contrary remark may be applied to warm water, as we have all experienced on getting out of a warm bath even in summer. A Russian lady of the author's acquaintance took a *warm* bath immediately after dinner, the result was, a want of reaction, and a complete paralysation of the whole of one side of the body.

Before entering cold water, we ought to wash the head and the chest, in order to prevent the blood ascending to those regions.

People, without knowing whether hot or mineral waters will be beneficial or otherwise, make use of them because it is the fashion so to do, or because their application is agreeable. A little reflection would show them that there will not be a wholesome reaction; that taken inwardly they must necessarily injure or destroy the coats of the stomach; and when applied outwardly, weaken the skin, thereby rendering the body susceptible to every change of weather.

Those who resort to sea-bathing in general pay little or no attention to diet. To derive advantage from a trip to any of our watering places, the latter, for the time at least, should be attended to.

The fact that the action of the human heart is repeated at least one hundred thousand times a-day, with sufficient force to keep in continual movement a mass of from 50 to 60 lbs. of blood, might lead to the inquiry what watch, what machinery could be more easily deranged? Can we wonder at men being ill who are constantly eating too much, who indulge in acid wines, in thick and adulterated beer, or spirituous liquors, or hot liquids of whatsoever nature they may be?

Few of us sufficiently appreciate pure cold water. What will not man submit to rather than adopt such means of cure—adapt himself to such self-denial? What pain will he not endure; what poisons swallow or rub into his flesh, rather than consent to seek relief from such a humble source?

Animals, when thirsty, repair to the brook to quench their thirst; when wounded, to assuage the pain. Water is nature's medicine and man despises it.

What organic matter can grow or live without water? We know that animals or plants excluded from its influence die. Observe the vivifying effects of water upon vegetation after a shower. Then what shall be said to vain, short-sighted man, who sets nature's laws at defiance, by avoiding what they enjoin, and indulging in what they interdict? Why should he live without water more than all else that has life? It may be answered "He does not live his time;" for every day's experience proves that more than half the inhabitants of the civilised world are tormented by one disease or another, which causes them to die before the natural term of life is completed. This, evidently, was not the intention of Divine Providence, since water, found every where, will prevent or cure disease, enable human beings to attain a good old age, and die without pain.

Stiffened joints, the dull eye, thickness of breathing, an unnatural tendency to corpulency, wrinkles, baldness, bad sight, and sallowness of complexion, are failings which clearly indicate an habitual distaste for water. It cannot be doubted, that in many of these cases, the mere drinking plentifully of water, and washing the body once a day, would afford relief. If they had always been accustomed to this they would not have been thus affected.

What numbers of weakly, crippled children we see? "Parents, do you wash their bodies; do you encourage them in the drinking of water? If not, you are instrumental to their future misery: you deprive them of the power of being healthy in life, or attaining to longevity." In looking around on the organic world, we cannot but admire the perfection everything seems to attain—the noblest work of creation an exception; we exclaim, with Goldsmith, "Man seems the only growth that dwindles here."

"Health is the natural state of man.

"The causes of bodily disease, not proceeding from external injury, are material, and consist of foreign matters introduced into the system.

"These foreign matters are divided into four parts:—

"I. Bodily substances which have not been eliminated in proper time.

"II. Substances not assimilated, and notwithstanding which, remain in the stomach, the skin, or the interior.

"Contagious ulcers.

"Corrupted elements; epidemical diseases.

"Every acute disease is an attempt to dispel diseased matter.

"Fever is not a disease, but the consequence of it; it is an effect of an exertion greater than the power of the system.

"The radical healing of acute diseases is only possible by releasing the diseased matter, by means of water, an agent which invariably effects its object, and that always in a manner perceptible to the senses.

"By means of physic and bleeding, acute diseases become chronic; the system, medically treated, effects a partial, but never a total ejection of diseased matter.

"As sooner or later a body must yield to the effects of drugs, it is quite impossible that any one suffering from chronic disease, unless healed by Hydropathy, should die a natural death.

"Chronic disease cannot be permanently cured by drugs: Hydropathy alone will effect this, by changing the chronic evil to acute eruptions, which are cured in the same way that acute diseases are cured.

"Men, like other organic beings, ought to live according to nature's law, without pain, and die a natural death, that is to say, without illness or suffering. But with us almost every body dies prematurely, from the effects of poisoning in some way or other."—ARBUTHNOT.

It was stated to Priessnitz, that in a case of gout, the bowels of the patient by the treatment, had become constipated, to which he replied, "Cold water never produces torpor of the bowels, but on the contrary, it excites."

"In the cure of disease, that which is most agreeable is not always the best. That which lowers the system, generally soothes and allays pain; bleeding, drugs, opium, and warm baths do this, but they may fix the disease firmer in the system, they diminish the energy so necessary to eradicate the disease. Thus Gout, Piles, and many other complaints, are never thoroughly cured by the faculty; they cannot abate the symptoms without lowering the system."

"To promote a crisis, dress lightly; warm clothing relaxes the skin. The stronger and harder the skin, the better will a crisis be developed. Every sore and boil cannot be considered a crisis, some degenerate into disease, and have an inward tendency. In a proper crisis of boils, they rise, burst, and heal."

"For itching rash in the arm, do not wear the bandage, unless great pain ensues, and in that case only at night."

"Chopping or sawing wood is better exercise for the stomach and bowels than walking."

To a lady who complained of want of sleep, and much pain from an eruption on her body, Priessnitz said "Take a tepid bath for some days, eat lean meat without salt, and indulge freely in butter, you will get well as soon as the rash has expended itself: there can be no repose for the nerves until the humours that fret them are expelled."

"Nervous temperaments are the strongest, but most irritable when excited by acid humours."

"Fingers being white after cold bathing denote weak nerves; the fingers having lost their vitality, the blood ceases to circulate."

"Constipation and relaxation of the bowels proceed from the same causes, weakness and impurities; hydropathy corrects both."

"It is impossible to warm, for any length of time, by hot viands and warm water, their constant application only chills the more; by relaxing and dilating they produce the opposite effects to those which are so essential to health, namely Contraction. Cold water determines the Caloric currents outwards from the vital centre, and promotes decomposition."

"I cannot understand how drugs can reach any destined point; it appears to me that all drugs are inimical to the human subject."

"Medicine introduced into the system, like the venom of a serpent, permeates all the tissues."

"Mercury becomes enveloped in phlegm or slime, and remains in the system, notwithstanding the body is continually subjected to the laws of renovation and decay."

"Powerful medicines act speedily and detrimentally to the constitution. The Water-cure is slow but advantageous in its operations."

"The wet sheet, which is in fact, a poultice, extracts pernicious matters, as a sponge water from a basin, and brings something away each time it is immersed in it."

XXXIII.—Questions put to Mr. Priessnitz, and his Answers.

1.—Q. What should be done for:—

Severe cold settled on the lungs, attended with cough and expectoration?

A. Rub the chest and throat with cold water, and hold water in the mouth often. In cold climates, bandage the throat: in warm climates, washing it often is best.

2.—Q. Inflammation and soreness of throat attended with hoarseness and difficulty in speaking?

A. As No. 1.

3.—Q. Exposure to change of climate with clothes occasionally wet, attended with shivering?

A. Rubbing-sheets.

4.—Q. Continual public speaking of damp evenings?

A. Rubbing-sheets. Wash head well. A foot-bath for a long time; and take exercise afterwards until feet are warm.

5.—Q. Cold accompanied by fever and restlessness at night?

A. As No. 4.

6.—Q. Head-ache occasioned by excitement?

A. As No. 4.

7.—Q. Shooting pain and tightness across the chest?

A. As No. 4, and rub the chest well with wet hand.

8.—Q. How guard against the effects of a damp atmosphere?

A. Keep the throat and chest always bare; if kept close and warm they will soon become relaxed. Parts most used should be exposed to the air.

9.—Q. At present I am packed for half an hour, and take the plunge bath at 5 A.M. Douche for three minutes at 12. Two Abreibungs and a Sitz-bath for half an hour at 5 P.M. If I remain the summer, should I continue or diminish this cure?

A. Continue it certainly for a month, and then begin to diminish it, leaving off the Douche for instance.

10.—Q. If continued, might I take the Douche after my walk in the morning before breakfast, and the Abreibungs at mid-day, so as to have my afternoons free?

A. Some cure must be taken after dinner as a rule; but in case of necessity the cure may be shirked.

11.—Q. Ought I to continue any part of the treatment on leaving Gräfenberg, and what?

A. Washing morning and evening, either bath or Abreibung.

12.—Q. After leaving must I attend to the same diet, and abstain entirely from Wine, Coffee, and Tea? or may I indulge in them continuously in small quantities, or only occasionally?

A. Wine, Coffee and Tea may be taken now and then, but by no means regularly.

13.—Q. On any return of my old complaints, blistered mouth, indigestion, restlessness, uneasy sensations in the back and side, what portion of the cure should I have recourse to?

A. The old complaints ought not to return, and will not if the cure is carried through the summer; on the appearance of any of them, they must be treated the same as they were here.

14.—Q. The sensations mentioned before now return sometimes; but vanish after a few days' severe treatment. It is only since the last month that my limbs and muscles have appeared to recover their tone and firmness, and enlarge.

A. Both of these observations speak volumes for the continuance of the cure, as one cannot do too much: but one may easily do too little; and it would be highly advisable to keep on cleansing and strengthening every possible way.

15.—Q. Should I continue any of the treatment for the child?

A. Bathe the child every morning and evening, that is, cold washing, by means of bath or Abreibungs.

16.—Q. Might I myself treat her in the cases of measles and scarlatina, and how?

A. In case of slight fever, a rubbing-sheet and Umschlag; but it is impossible to prescribe beforehand how these diseases are to be treated, as one cannot know how the child may be affected. If the fever is severe, more wet sheets or rubbing-sheets must be used than if it is slight. The criterion of treatment is the degree of fever.

TREATMENT AND CASES.

XXXIV.—Gout.

Great difference of opinion exists as to the cause of gout. Ancient physicians called it the daughter of Bacchus and Venus; and truly persons, or their progeny, devoted to these two divinities, offer the greatest number of examples.

To cure this complaint, the ingenuity of thousands of scientific men has been taxed, and the whole pharmacopœia applied to in vain. Perspiration is mostly resorted to; but as this is effected by warm baths, vapour baths, or drugs, the consequences are so debilitating that few constitutions can bear them. The result of all medical treatment in this disease is, the degradation of robust constitutions, and the promotion of diseases worse than the gout itself.

Volumes might be written on the various remedial measures which have been resorted to in this complaint, and of which time has shewn the fallacy. We now ask the invalid, if he ever knew the gout radically cured by any pharmaceutical means? Were Hydropathists asked whether they ever knew cases of gout cured by water, they would unhesitatingly answer in the affirmative. Incipient gout is always curable. The same may be said of chronic gout, except in isolated cases: then Hydropathy invariably gives relief; and by regulating the functions of the body, improves the general health.

The following treatment and cases will shew how the manipulation is varied, to combat this disease in its manifold forms:—

Gout cannot be cured by local applications; the whole system must be purified by a general treatment, or no permanent cure can be effected.

For occasional attacks of gout in the extremities, the constitution being otherwise robust:—

In the morning, put a bandage on the part affected, pack the patient in blankets (sweating process) until perspiration appears in the face.

Then put him into the half-bath—water 62° to 65° Fahr.; let him be well rubbed in this from 5 to 25 minutes, or until friction can be applied to all parts alike. Cold water should be occasionally poured over head and shoulders during the operation. This ended, put bandages round the waist and on the afflicted part.

For the second treatment:—About mid-day, rubbed in a packing-sheet; take a sitz-bath for fifteen minutes—first time tepid 64°, afterwards cold; then put the offending member into cold water for ten or fifteen minutes, and renew bandages.

In the afternoon, at 5 o'clock, repeat mid-day treatment. During the day, drink ten to fourteen tumblers of water.

The above treatment will generally put an end to a slight attack of gout; but to eradicate it from the system, the cure must be followed up. To effect this, for the sweating process on the second day, substitute the packing-sheet until warm, which generally requires the patient to lie in it from thirty minutes to an hour.

Where a bath cannot be obtained, the rubbing sheet is used instead; this should be very little wrung out, and if one does not cool the body, a second or a third should be applied.

The douche is often applied in gout; but as that cannot be the case in ordinary practice, the practitioner must use his discretion in prescribing it.

It is good treatment to use the sweating process in the morning, and the packing-sheet in the afternoon.

The bandages must be worn day and night, and changed often.

Cases.—A patient, fifty years of age, with rheumatic gout, bad digestion, nervousness, fingers blue and swollen, slight pain in the knee, much debilitated, was ordered:—In the morning, five rubbing sheets, two or three minutes each, allowing a short interim between each. At noon, the same. At five o'clock, the same. Ten tumblers of water daily. Bandages to parts affected, and round the loins always. On the patient experiencing great pain under the knees, the morning treatment was changed to lying in packing-sheets until well warmed, followed by the tepid bath. Patient soon improved in health.

A——, forty-six years of age, suffered fifteen years from periodical attacks of gout, and had his last severe attack in his feet, hands, and elbows, accompanied by paralysis, which affected his voice.

Treatment.—Laid in packing-sheet until perspiration ensued (two or three hours); then tepid bath renewed by cold water being thrown over head and shoulders; noon, rubbing-sheet, followed by sitz-bath 62° for fifteen minutes; cold foot-bath fifteen minutes, and head-bath ten minutes; afternoon, morning treatment repeated.

Alternate days, sweating in blankets instead of the sheets; all other treatment the same as before.

This continued treatment was persevered in for ten weeks, when patient was prescribed sweating in the morning, and packing-sheet in the afternoon, followed by cold bath. Sitz and foot-baths as before; head-bath discontinued. Shortly after, sweating twice a day, with foot-baths, fifteen minutes in the middle of the day. Sitz-baths dispensed with. This treatment at the end of six weeks was again changed for perspiring only once a day, for three hours. Patient was at length ordered to discontinue the treatment altogether, and proceed to the sea-side for a month. Soon after his return again to Gräfenberg, he was able to walk fifteen miles at a time, as is seen by his own letter.

B——, fifty-six years of age, suffering from Gout upwards of seventeen years, generally incapacitated from following his occupation seven or eight months in a year. Feet and hands distorted.

Treatment.—Packing sheet and tepid-bath in morning and afternoon, and sitz and foot-bath, each fifteen minutes; at noon, bandages round the waist. After a week's treatment, a fit of gout came on in foot and ankle, which was combated by packing-sheet and tepid bath before breakfast; tepid sitz-bath at noon, and the morning treatment repeated in the afternoon. After three days, a boil began to form under the left jaw; treatment continued, with the exception of patient's going (*after the packing-sheet*), into tepid bath for two minutes, then into the cold bath for two minutes, and back to the tepid, from ten to fifteen minutes.

In eight days, gout returned with greater violence, when recourse was had to the packing-sheet, as before; with tepid baths from twenty minutes to an hour, besides following up other parts of the treatment. In seven or eight days the fit quite subsided. Some time after this he had a relapse, which patient stated to me, under the allopathic treatment, would have confined him to his room at least six months; this was treated as follows:—

Packing-sheet until warm, followed by tepid bath, ten minutes; then walked about the room for a quarter of an hour; then the bath again for a quarter of an hour, a respite of a few minutes, and the bath a third time.

Two hours after the above operation, a tepid sitting-bath 62°, for twenty minutes.

In the afternoon the packing-sheet and bath as before. This treatment was repeated, every day for six days, when patient was out of doors again.

From this time patient felt himself so changed a man, that the author saw him cry with joy. He could use his limbs as he had not done for many years, and to prove it, ran up a hill with astonishing alacrity. Three days treatment were sufficient to reduce the swelling of his knuckles, toes, and hands.

This patient, on his first arrival, Mr. Priessnitz ordered, without any previous preparation, into a tepid bath, where he was rubbed upwards of an hour.

C——, aged forty. Gout generally returned in summer.

Treatment.—Morning, and afternoon, packing-sheet, tepid bath; noon, douche, three minutes.

After six weeks treatment, strong redness and much pain to the conjunctiva; douche omitted.

Sitz-baths of from an hour to an hour and a half; foot-baths; cold wet bandages to the eye, which became effected.

Then sweating processes, with wet bandages to the head, which afforded relief.

Alternate tepid, cold and tepid baths for a quarter of an hour; immediately after the packing-sheet, foot-bath and water poured over the ancle. Eyes still red; foot-bath resorted to three times a day, followed by rubbing sheet, instead of the bath and bandage to the eye. Eyes could bear the light. Patient's appetite good and sleep sound. At night his arms, head, and most of his body were covered with bandages.

In three weeks, patient's whole body covered with an eruption; recourse again had to the packing-sheet and tepid bath twice a day. From this time health improved daily.

D——, a gouty subject, forty-five years of age. Priessnitz, called up in the middle of the night, found the Baron labouring under an attack of gout in his chest and stomach, which almost prevented his breathing. He was immediately put into a packing-sheet for from five to ten minutes, and out of that into a tepid bath, where two men rubbed him for a quarter of an hour; cold water being continually thrown over his head and shoulders; this effectually put an end to the attack, and the patient afterwards slept soundly until the time for his usual treatment next morning. This case shows that the fear of this treatment driving gout to the stomach, is groundless and it combats a dangerous attack, and quicker than it can be done by any other means.

Hereditary Gout.—E——, a Polish nobleman, fifty-four years of age, suffered two winters from hereditary gout, which had existed in his family for upwards of forty years.

He was attacked in his feet and arms, which confined him to his bed several months.

Treatment:—In the mornings, packing-sheet and tepid bath; noon, rubbing-sheet followed by sitz-bath, fifteen minutes; afternoon, rubbing-sheet.

In eighteen days he had boils on his feet and arms, from which matter continued to exude for three or four weeks; at the expiration of which Priessnitz said, "Now we will increase the treatment, to see if any more bad matter remains in the system."

The sweating process and cold bath were now resorted to three or four times a week; the packing-sheet and cold bath other days; and the douche every day for three minutes. This treatment was continued for several weeks, during which no change of any kind was produced, a confirmation of the cure being effected.

On leaving Gräfenberg, Priessnitz advised him to return the next year, to see if the cure was a radical one.

In 1845, the Count returned, when he was subjected to a most vigorous treatment, such as sweating, douche, etc., for a month, without any return of gout.

On leaving Gräfenberg he assured me, that he was not only cured of gout; but that his digestive powers, which for years had been deranged, were in perfect order, and that his general health was completely restored.

Sixteen years previous to the Count's going to Gräfenberg, he had his elbow wounded by a ball in a duel, which occasionally caused him great pain. For the cure of this, he, at the time, rubbed in a yellow ointment. Singular to say, after a lapse of sixteen years, during a crisis, this ointment re-appeared on the elbow and arm, so thick as to be taken off with the finger. The exuding of this ointment lasted about eight days. Since the cure of his gout was effected, the arm has been pliant, and the elbow has been free from pain.

Gout in Head and Feet.—F——, a German professor, aged sixty; a small delicate man, with gout in both hands and both feet: all were contracted, he had been a martyr to gout for years and upwards, when a paroxysm of gout came on the following morning.

The following treatment was resorted to. Morning, packing-sheet until thoroughly warm; then tepid bath 64° for two hours, during which time 200 cans of cold water were thrown over his head and shoulders.

Twenty-five cans were first thrown; then great friction for some time; then twenty-five cans more, followed by friction; and so repeated until two hundred cans had been thrown over him.

Heating bandages were applied to all parts afflicted, and kept there day and night.

The above treatment was resorted to again in the afternoon.

One paroxysm that I witnessed, lasted three weeks. It was astonishing to see the courage displayed by this patient.

Each operation afforded relief for the time; but the enemy had strong hold upon the system, and was ejected with difficulty.

During all the time the patient had a good appetite and slept soundly at night.

He was still under the cure when I left Gräfenberg. Priessnitz said, to effect this cure, it would require at least four years' treatment, which the patient said he would prefer to a renewal of the suffering he had already undergone, previously to coming to Gräfenberg.

Calcareous Deposit in the Knees, and high state of Inflammation.—The last case shews how the human body may be exposed to the action of water, with friction, for any length of time. The present case is that of an English Gentleman, well known to all visitors at Gräfenberg.

G——, aged between 50 and 60, gouty for the last twenty years, with contraction of the limbs, chalk stones having formed in the joints. This patient travelled from Italy to Gräfenberg during the heat of summer, and, on arriving, had a most painful attack of gout in his lower extremities.

Priessnitz, without the least preparation, put him into a tepid bath, and he was rubbed by three men for nearly three hours, occasionally throwing pails of cold water over his head and shoulders. This so reduced the inflammation, that, towards the end of that period, the afflicted part might also be rubbed with the wet hand.

Heating bandages were then applied to those parts and the waist.

Water was drunk plentifully during and after the operation.

Patient was able afterwards to get out of doors with the use of sticks, and slept well at night.

Next morning he began the regular treatment, which was as follows:—

Packing-sheet until warm; then the bath as before for about two hours; noon, rubbing-sheet and sitz-bath, fifteen minutes; afternoon, morning process renewed.

Mr. Priessnitz told this patient that, by the following means, he might always ward off a violent attack of gout:—

On feeling the slightest sensation of gout, he should instantly be put into a tepid bath, 62 deg., replenished with cold water, and be therein rubbed for a couple of hours.

This gentleman's general health is perfect: he very seldom has any attacks, and they are slight; but the calcareous deposit in his knees, up to the present, resists all attempts at removal.

Acute attack of Gout.—A patient being attacked with gout was put into a tepid bath, 68 deg., up to the neck, and rubbed by himself and two men. By particular injunctions, the process was not to be discontinued until all pain subsided. The original temperature of the bath was maintained by fresh supplies of cold water. In seven hours the patient was completely relieved. His after-treatment was:—

Morning, packing-sheet and plunge-bath, bandage round the waist and on part afflicted; at noon, douche, and afterwards a rubbing-sheet; afternoon, rubbing-sheet; the simplest food. On a return of the acute attack, patient was ordered to perform the bath operation again; but, not persevering in remaining seven hours in the bath, the attack was not overcome: the patient was then ordered cold bath every morning before breakfast (temperature kept always as cold as possible), from fifteen to twenty minutes, which effected the cure. This patient was allowed a little weak chocolate, and was ordered to drink abundantly of water.

A—— had a most violent attack at Gräfenberg, for which he was put up to his neck into a tepid bath, 64 deg., and there rubbed by two men for *seven* hours. Priessnitz gave particular orders that the patient should not leave the bath until all pain had completely subsided. Cold water was frequently added, to keep that in the bath at the original temperature. By these means the attack was completely subdued. Daily treatment:—

Morning, packing-sheet and cold plunge-bath; bandage to be applied to parts affected; noon, douche, and sitz-bath, fifteen minutes; afternoon, as in the morning.

Instructions:—Eat plain food; and in case of a return of gout, faithfully perform the first operation.

Gout in the Foot and Ankle.—A lady awoke in the morning with pain in her foot and ankle, which were both swollen.

Treatment.—Packing-sheet for an hour, followed by a rubbing-sheet; after which a foot-bath, up to the instep, for a quarter of an hour; and the foot and leg, up to the knee, well rubbed all the time.

Bandages were then applied from the toes to the knee.

At noon, and in the afternoon, the foot-bath was again applied, and the bandages were changed.

This simple treatment put an end to the attack in two days. If it had not done so, it ought to have been repeated.

XXXV.—RHEUMATISM, ETC.

Gout, rheumatism, sciatica, lumbago, tic douloureux, and neuralgia, all being attended with inflammation, are so nearly allied, that the same treatment as for gout, with slight variation, might be applied to any or all of them.

Rheumatism.—On a slight attack of rheumatism, rub the part affected with wet hands three times a day, from a quarter of an hour to an hour each time; then apply a bandage, which change when dry, and wear it until the pain ceases.

Rub the body all over with a wet towel, then a dry one; wait five minutes, then repeat the same operation four times in succession: this will animate the circulation. Then apply a bandage as in the case of gout. This treatment should be applied several times a day. Rheumatic subjects ought never to be overclothed, wear flannel, or fail drinking water.

When the attack is more severe, three rubbing-sheets in succession, allowing an interim of from three to five minutes between each. The body must be dried after each rubbing-sheet; this increases the effect of the next rubbing-sheet. Rub the parts affected often with wet hands, and apply bandages. This treatment may be repeated three or four times a day. If there is a great want of circulation, the patient may lie in bed until warm, between the application of each rubbing-sheet.

Neuralgic Pains.—Whatever the nature of these pains may be (supposing the patient not too debilitated), perspiration will generally be found to relieve them. To effect this:—

When in bed in the morning, add a number of blankets, and on them a feather-bed: there remain until in a profuse perspiration; then cool the body, either by rubbing-sheets, a cold bath,—or get a washing-tub, stand up in it, and have some jugs of water poured over the head and shoulders. This very often settles the affair at once.

A patient was afflicted in every joint so that he could not be moved in bed without great pain.

Packing-sheets until warm, which required about half an hour, ten times a day, allowing an interval between them. Each packing sheet was followed by a rubbing with wet hands.

This treatment in one day enabled patient to stand; then the packing sheets were used four times a day, followed by rubbing sheets. Parts affected and loins always enclosed in bandages. Patient drank sixteen to twenty glasses of water a day. He was out of doors the third day, and afterwards pursued a more vigorous treatment, such as sweating, douche, &c.

A——, had a severe rheumatic attack in both knees; he thought swinging his legs backwards and forwards would relieve him; instead of which, it brought on enlargement of the joints and inflammation: whilst at Gräfenberg I inquired of Priessnitz what he ought to have done.—

Answer—He ought in, the first instance, to have rubbed the knees well and often with wet hands and worn a bandage. If this was not sufficient, then to have put the feet and legs, over the knees into cold water for half an hour at least, rubbing them all the time, and apply a bandage from the calf of the leg to the middle of the thigh.

Chronic Rheumatism.—A——, contracted rheumatism in 1837, which commenced as sciatica. Constitution greatly debilitated. Medical advice, sea baths, hot baths, and other remedies, useless.

Patient went to Gräfenberg, August 1843, and left in May following.

Treatment.—Packing-sheet, followed by cold bath twice a-day; noon, sitz-bath and foot-bath, fifteen minutes each; legs rubbed all the time up to the knee. Douche three minutes daily.

In November, one of his usual attacks came on, when sixteen rubbing sheets a-day were resorted to. Four of these were given in succession four times a-day; between each rubbing sheet, the patient being weak lay down in bed, until warm bandages were applied as usual.

This attack subsided after the second day, when patient renewed his former treatment.

B——, travelling in North America, and exposed to severe rains without the means of changing his clothes, suffered the consequences such circumstances frequently entail. Rheumatism almost beyond endurance induced him to go to Gräfenberg.

At the first interview, Priessnitz put him first into a tepid bath 64 deg., out of which he plunged into a cold bath, where he staid about a minute, and from that he returned again to the tepid, when bandages were applied to his waist and parts affected.

Treatment.—Morning, packing-sheet until warm, then cold bath; noon, rubbing-sheet; afternoon, packing-sheet, twenty minutes, and then rubbing-sheet again.

Left Gräfenberg in a month, during which time patient used the rubbing-sheet mornings and evenings; exposed his body (after that in the morning) quite naked in his room, from a quarter to half an hour.

On returning to Gräfenberg, the douche was substituted for the rubbing-sheet at noon. After continuing the treatment for some time, rheumatism returned, when he was ordered three rubbing-sheets five minutes each, twice a-day; between each an air bath of five minutes.

A crisis of boils ensued, and after they healed, patient was perfectly well. The patient writes to a friend—"I now leave Gräfenberg with a clean body, and a sincere wish for your own speedy cure, and that of all the agreeable acquaintances that I leave behind me, under the safe care of our virtuous and sagacious friend V. Priessnitz."

Chronic Rheumatism, Chronic Headache, Constipation, Piles, &c.—A Gentleman, aged about 45, was treated as follows:—

Morning, sweating process and cold bath, three minutes; noon, douche, three minutes; an hour afterwards, sitz-bath fifteen minutes; foot-bath fifteen minutes; head-bath ten minutes; one following the other immediately; afternoon, noon treatment over again; all night—loins, feet, legs, and thighs, to the fork, were encased in bandages.

In a few months, rheumatism, piles, and constipation were cured, but headache returned at intervals.

Rheumatic attack in the Back, Shoulders, and Neck.—The sweating process, followed by three rubbing-sheets not much wrung out, applied without intermission for five minutes each, put an end to the attack at once. If this number of rubbing-sheets had not cooled the body, more must have been used.

Had rheumatism continued, rubbing-sheets must have been resorted to again in the afternoon, and the sweating resumed the next day.

Rheumatic Fever.—For a slight attack of rheumatic fever, three rubbing-sheets three times a-day were found sufficient.

Rheumatic Gout.—A gentleman named Heymann, about 34 years of age, at the fire at Hamburg was exposed to the wet from the engines for several days and nights. The result was, a violent attack of rheumatic gout; first in the knees and feet, then neck and arms; afterward in hip and both breasts, which confined him to bed a whole year, from April 1843 to April 1844.

During this time he took large quantities of medicine, and used steam and sulphur baths: about seventy of the former, and near a hundred of the latter. Also mud and sulphur baths, which enabled him to walk for about a month, when he was again confined to bed. Gout having attacked the breast, both his medical attendants declared they could do no more. 1st May, 1844, he was conveyed to Gräfenberg, so crippled that he could not dress himself. He began the treatment as follows:—

Morning, packing-sheet and tepid bath; noon, three rubbing-sheets, at intervals of five minutes, with open windows; afternoon, packing-sheet one hour, and tepid bath; bandage round the body, and from ankles to knees during the night.

Pain increasing, parts affected were rubbed with wet hands both day and night until they became hot. Body entirely bandaged by night. Bandage changed three or four times as pain resulted from the bandages being dry.

At the expiration of three months, patient enabled to walk out. Treatment changed.

Morning, packing-sheet and tepid bath; noon, one rubbing-sheet, followed by sitz-bath for quarter of an hour; douche before and after breakfast for three minutes; then morning and evening packing-sheet and bath; tepid for two minutes; then cold one minute and back to tepid bath for two minutes, instead of an entire tepid bath.

Two months' continuation of this treatment brought out an eruption around the body, and on the calves of the legs; also a strong fever which lasted nine days, which was succeeded by boils.

Then three packing-sheet a-day were applied, and tepid, cold, and tepid baths; continually changing from one to another for an hour and a half. Douche and rubbing-sheet stopped during the fever.

The eruption continued for three months, discharging whitish brown matter. During all this time the last treatment was persevered in.

The eruption and boils gave great relief. When pain was diminished and the eruption ceased, the body bandage was relinquished and those of the waist and calves retained, and cold bath for one minute, succeeded the packing sheet.

1st April, 1845. Douche, from three to five minutes, substituted for the rubbing-sheet.

May 16th, 1845.—Patient was declared perfectly well. He had gone the whole of the winter without stockings, neckcloth, or waistcoat, wearing only linen coat and trousers, and sleeping with his windows wide open. When I saw him at Gräfenberg, in May, I thought I never saw a man in such robust rude health in my life.

This case made a great sensation at Hamburg, as the party is well known on the exchange of that city.

Sciatica.—A soldier aged 35, after having been three months in the hospital with Sciatica, without relief, was cured in five days by the following treatment:—

In the morning sweating process and cold bath; noon, two rubbing-sheets; afternoon, the same; much rubbing at other times with wet hands. Bandages to the part were applied, and much water drank.

This case was treated by the author at Limerick; and the following process was adopted:—

Sciatica and Lumbago.—Patient ordered:—Morning, four rubbing-sheets; at noon, the same; afternoon the same, and if necessary, to be repeated on going to bed. The usual interval of time between each sheet to be observed, and parts affected covered in bandages. The treatment to have been repeated next day, had not the first removed the pains.

In all cases of this nature, Rubbing with wet hands is highly beneficial, and sometimes Enemas of cold water should be resorted to. If obstinate, the sweating process must be employed. I knew a very severe acute case of Sciatica and Lumbago relieved in two days, by the application of four rubbing-sheets at four intervals during the day, and the evening bandages were applied, and water drunk in abundance.

Lumbago or Rick in the Back.—A young man woke early in the morning with a most excruciating pain in his loins. He could not determine whether it was simply Lumbago, or a Rick in the back, brought on from playing at skittles or chopping wood the day before.

Priessnitz had him turned on his stomach, his back rubbed for an hour with wet hands, and then covered with a bandage.

The Rubbing was to be repeated every four hours, and the bandage changed every two hours.

The patient was to remain lying on his stomach the whole day and night if not cured. The reason for this must be evident to those who reflect upon it. Cured the same day.

Violent attack of Lumbago, supposed to have been brought on by using the dumb-bells; the party being unaccustomed to their use.

Patient had rubbing with wet hands, and wearing a bandage for two days, when he could hardly rise from a chair; then he commenced the following treatment:—

Saturday.—Morning, packing-sheet for an hour, followed by three rubbing-sheets; noon, two rubbing-sheets and an Enema; night, a rubbing-sheet. This was not renewed at night, as patient's extremities were cold and prevented his sleeping.

Sunday.—Four rubbing-sheets; after this operation, the improvement was almost miraculous. Patient took a long walk.

Monday.—Treatment as yesterday; could turn in bed with less difficulty.

Tuesday.—Packing-sheet forty minutes, preceded by a tepid-bath sixteen minutes, with great friction; noon, four rubbing-sheets; evening, loins rubbed with wet hands for half-an-hour.

Wednesday.—Slept well and could turn with ease in bed; three rubbing-sheets and friction thrice during the day with wet hands.

Drank fourteen tumblers of water daily, and wore a bandage night and day.

Thursday.—Perfectly well. By the means here described, patient's bowels were kept in order; his tongue always clean. Had his treatment failed, the sweating process must have been resorted to.

XXXVI.—Tic-Doloureux.

This is another of those complaints that baffle medical skill, and upon which medical men are at issue as to the cause; some alleging it to be a derangement of the nervous system, others think it is in the humours of the body, which contain an acrimony irritating to the nerves.

The result of my observation is, that if under the Water cure, it is not cured in three months, it is extremely doubtful if it will succumb to that treatment. Dr. Munde doubted if purely nervous Tic-doloureux was curable by any process; but speaks more positively as to that which arises from acrimonious humour. He says, "I speak with a perfect knowledge of this disease, having suffered for three years, and having made observations upon several others who suffered severely from this complaint. Eight months' treatment cured me after trying all other remedies in vain."

I knew a patient who had laboured under Tic in his head for fourteen or fifteen years, perfectly cured in three months. His treatment was the same as for Rheumatism.

Another patient put a bandage to her face at night, whilst under a paroxysm of Tic; this increased the pain, the reason of which was, her not having prepared the system first. Next day she underwent the sweating process, and could then wear the bandage with great advantage.

A person, whom I knew, suffering from Tic in his legs, made no progress because of the injudicious use of the Douche. The Douche was abandoned, and the packing-sheet and tepid bath twice a day substituted with great advantage.

Another *case of severe* Tic came under my notice, that resisted all treatment. The paroxysm was only allayed by very long tepid baths 62°, and great friction.

Obstinate case of Tic in the Thigh.—This case is given to shew the way in which Priessnitz meets extraordinary circumstances.

H. from Berlin, aged 54, had a settled pain down one of his thighs; he was treated for it seven years ago at Gräfenberg. In a few months he thought himself cured. For seven years he felt no inconvenience, and lived as he had formerly done. At the expiration of that period, pain returned; not wishing to devote so much time to the cure as he knew it would require at

Gräfenberg, he went to Carlsbad, where the pain became insupportable. In this state he again had recourse to Priessnitz. He has now been there four months, undergoing a vigorous treatment of packing-sheets, baths, rubbing-sheets, and sitz-baths, varied in an infinity of ways, without experiencing much benefit; his sleep, which has been disturbed the last eighteen months, still continues so.

Nearly all the sleep he obtains is in the packing-sheet. In this he lies from his arm-pits down to his thighs, from 9 to 11 o'clock at night, and again from 2 to 4 o'clock in the morning. At 6 o'clock he commences his usual treatment. The last fortnight before I left Gräfenberg, pain had ceased, but his sleeping was as disturbed as usual.

XXXVII.—Affection of the Throat and Pain at the Chest.

A delicate lady, aged twenty-five: morning, packing-sheet until warm and tepid bath; noon, rubbing-sheet and sitz-bath; afternoon, rubbing-sheet.

After a few days' treatment, catamenia came on, notwithstanding which, as patient experienced no inconvenience, the treatment was continued as before. In two days, pain in the abdomen and hips was felt. All the previous treatment was now discontinued, and three rubbing-sheets a day were prescribed, until pain ceased, when it was again resumed.

Throat, and pain at the chest, were cured in six weeks, and patient had gained eight pounds in weight.

This lady thought she had an affection of the heart. Priessnitz enquired if she felt pain there: she answered no. "Then," said he, "the heart is sound." Three years ago, catamenia lasted only five days, but latterly it extended to seven. Priessnitz said, with her it ought only to last three or four days. This was effected. Her husband, who had occasional attacks of bile, gained nine pounds in six weeks. I attended the weighing of these parties, and can vouch for the fact.

XXXVIII.—Fevers.

Two Hundred Years Ago, Dr. Vanderheyden of Ghent wrote a work in which he declared all fevers curable by cold water. Dr. Sir John Floyer, fifty years later, wrote his work, and then came Drs. Hahn, Smith and others, and finally, Dr. Currie of Liverpool, who by their works supported the same theory. It is true that though where medicine saved its hundreds, their practice saved thousands, the *Modus Operandi* was somewhat speculative. It was reserved until our own time to witness the application of water reduced to a science. Priessnitz by his packing-sheet has produced the great desideratum, which renders his treatment omnipotent over all febrile disorders; and if he had discovered nothing else, this would hand his name down to the latest posterity.

It is often asked what fevers are curable by the Hydropathic processes. To this it may be answered, except where by age or disease patients are not reduced to the last stage of existence, *all* are curable. I made constant inquiries when at Gräfenberg—witnessed the treatment of innumerable cases of fever, amongst others Typhus and Brain Fever, and I could not discover that Priessnitz during his long practice had ever lost a patient.

I have frequently treated cases of fever and inflammation myself with the most heartfelt satisfaction; as in every instance on the application of the sheet or the bath, the patient was relieved in the same manner that a plant dying for the want of water, is resuscitated on being supplied with it.

After the number of works published on this subject, all protesting the safety of this mode of treatment, and the total absence of danger, it may be fairly presumed, that the packing-sheet process will ere long take the lead in medical practice.

As almost all complaints trace their origin to fever or inflammation, if these can be allayed on their first symptoms, a host of evils to the human family will be avoided.

It does not require any great sagacity to perceive that when the body is surcharged with heat, if enveloped in a damp sheet, the sheet immediately becomes hot; take it away and you remove with it a certain amount of heat. The oftener this is repeated the more the calorie is diminished, and each sheet requires more time to heat; continue changing the sheet, and the body resumes a normal state. When once the heat is eliminated the patient is cured of the Fever.

The following modes of treatment and cases will enable the practitioner to judge how he should treat his patient as circumstances may arise.

As general rules:—

In the cold fit, use rubbing-sheets well wrung out, with a slight interim between each until the hot stage is produced. In the hot stage packing-sheets should be changed as often as necessary. In Typhus I have known them changed forty or fifty times in a day. The bath which ought at first to be a little tepid and cooled by degrees, should be resorted to at intervals twice or thrice a day, from a quarter of an hour to an hour. Should the heat action be prematurely violent, or likely to end in inflammation, resort to a sitz-bath with or without a foot-bath, instead of the tepid bath, particularly where either the brain, organs of sense, or those within the thorax are at all engaged.

Rubbing-sheets, in certain cases where the vital energies are weak or languid, will be sufficient to suppress a febrile paroxysm. Their renewal and time of application must entirely depend on the age, strength and idiosyncrasy of the case: water should be drunk in small quantities, and frequently.

Where the brain is attacked, water must be constantly applied to that locality, so as not to allow of an increase of temperature.

Where there is no want of bodily strength in the patient, the quickest and surest method of putting an end at once to fever, is as follows. Put him into a bath up to the shoulders, tepid 63° or 64° to begin with, and to be renewed constantly by cold water being poured over the shoulders; two persons rubbing the patient the whole time.

When he is quite fatigued, take him out, dry the body and throw the window open for air; when recovered a little, renew the operation, and so on for the third time if necessary. Then dress and go out to walk. Drink plentifully of water.

If very cold on coming out of the bath, walk without the body bandage, but put a large thick one from the hips to the arm-pits on returning home. Let the patient rest two or three hours; and if fever return repeat the foregoing treatment.

A Mr. B——, who was greatly debilitated, had, for fever, a tepid bath for half an hour to an hour and half; also many rubbing-sheets; on one occasion as many as twenty-nine in a day. If the fever resist the above treatment, then resort to the packing-sheet.

Dr. L——, for fever, ordered, five or six rubbing-sheets in succession. Head bath for a quarter of an hour. Bandage from hips to arm-pits, to be changed often, even in the night; to be much in the open air.

In typhus fever, medical men do not make the distinction between congestion of the venous and arterial systems. They imagine that inflammatory action exists, whereas it is in typhus, venous congestion: therefore, the leeching and severe depletory measures are decidedly wrong; they increase the existing evil, lower and exhaust the vital powers, and if persevered in, lead to death, or a long lingering state of convalescence. On the contrary, Hydropathy acts upon a diametrically opposite system: by the imbibition of water, containing as it does an excess of oxygen, the vital forces are sustained, the blood is decarbonised, the appetite improved, the bowels regulated, etc. etc.

Fever.—An English officer who caught a fever twenty years ago in the West Indies, wrote to Priessnitz that all his prospects in life were blighted, and that existence was almost intolerable. He came to Gräfenberg and was treated as follows:

Early in the morning packing-sheet and bath; wore heating bandage always. Breakfasted at eight o'clock, when, from nine o'clock until five o'clock in the evening, he was ordered to change the waist bandage every ten minutes. At five o'clock packing-sheet and bath.

If ague appeared, which it did sometimes, then rubbing-sheets, well wrung out were applied with great friction until the fit was over.

This patient was perfectly cured in three months.

Nervousness and slow Fever, and disposition to a Decline.—A lady was treated as follows:—

Morning, five packing-sheets and bath, 62°; noon, douche and sitz-bath; afternoon, rubbing-sheet and two sitz-baths.

At first, she was ordered to have a cold bath prepared by the bed-side at night, and when fever and sweating came on, to go into the bath, and repeat it if necessary. She had a bad cough at the time; her friends thought such a proceeding would end in her death; the patient, however, recovered from her fever and cough, and left much improved in health.

On awaking in the morning with distracting head-ache, parched tongue, and all the concomitants of fever, a lady was put into a packing-sheet; in twelve minutes, head-ache ceased. After remaining enveloped an hour or two, rubbing-sheets were applied, followed by a sitz-bath of twenty minutes: she drank water freely. This one application effected a cure.

A young lady had her foot and ankle much swollen from rheumatic gout. Second day, arose with head-ache and pain in all her limbs; and towards evening, had a slight fever. For this, she was put into a tepid bath 62°, and rubbed for forty minutes, when the arm-pits feeling no warmer than the other parts of her body, she was allowed to leave the bath. This application was sufficient.

Typhus Fever requires the same treatment as other fevers. The packing-sheet must be changed every ten or fifteen minutes: I have known it changed as much as fifty times a day. When the patient is weary of lying in the packing-sheet, he should be put into a tepid bath and well rubbed for a time; and then lie quiet, with a packing-sheet doubled several times from hips to arm-pits. Then packing-sheets should be resorted to again. If the head is attacked, apply the head-bath whilst lying in packing-sheet. Drink abundantly of water.

Packing sheets, tepid baths, and cold baths (the former often repeated), are also the treatment for brain fever. When a patient was in a state of delirium,

Priessnitz ordered her into a cold bath for an hour.

Teething fever.—Tepid head-bath—water gradually made colder—applied to the back of the head for half an hour.

If this had not had the desired effect it was to have been repeated after a short interval. Heating-bandages were to have been applied from the hips to the arm-pits.

Gastric Fever.—A young man attacked with gastric fever, was treated as follows:—

Two packing-sheets, one after the other, until warm, followed, by tepid bath, in which he was rubbed fifteen minutes, then put into cold bath for one minute, and from that back again to the tepid bath for fifteen minutes; patient was then dried, waited a few minutes, and then the bathing as above was twice repeated.

The whole of the treatment, *i. e.* packing sheet and baths, was repeated three times during the day; between which, a sitz-bath of half an hour was prescribed.

Patient was cured in two days, and then declared himself stronger and better than he was previously to the attack.

A gentleman aged thirty-four was thus treated:—

Packing-sheets twice a day until warm, followed by tepid bath.

Two sitz-baths a day, twenty minutes each. Patient's back, shoulders, abdomen and chest to be rubbed the whole time whilst taking the sitting-baths.

Patient having lost his appetite, Priessnitz recommended him to eat plentifully of common unripe plums: these deranged his stomach, of which he was immediately cured; and afterwards his appetite was better.

My servant was seized with violent pains in the abdomen during the night, and in the morning head-ache and fever. Dr. Farr of Nice, who saw the case, said depletion was requisite, and that the man might be well in four or five days. I declared with Hydropathy he might be made to wait at table the same day. He was put into a packing-sheet for an hour and a half, then a bath; an hour afterwards a sitz-bath; wore the bandage and required no further treatment. Dr. F——, until the next morning could not believe that the fever was subdued.

Capt. D—— ordered, in the morning, two packing-sheets until warm, with head in a basin of cold water all the time; followed by tepid bath, renewed with cold; noon, cold sitz-bath one hour; afternoon, morning treatment repeated.

Bilious Fever.—A female attacked with bilious fever, swelled face, and violent tooth-ache. Patient in the first instance, preferred consulting a medical man, who administered a strong aperient; ordered the feet to be kept in a hot bath for an hour, and said the fever would certainly last seven days, if not longer.

I applied a packing-sheet, and changed it after twenty minutes; then two rubbing-sheets. Head-bath 62° for a quarter of an hour: hot-water poultice to face. This treatment completely subdued the fever the second day.

Patient attacked with bilious fever, swelled face, and violent tooth-ache.

Packing-sheet for twenty, and another for thirty minutes; then two rubbing-sheets, twice a day; head-bath 62°, and sitz-bath 62°; hot water bandage to face.

On a return of the same in the spring of the next year: morning, packing-sheet and rubbing-sheet; noon, sitz-bath 62°; afternoon, sitz-bath and foot-bath 62°; the swollen part of the face put into cold water fifteen minutes, twice a day. This treatment answered admirably.

Nervous Fever.—Commencement of patient's illness was attended with violent headache and excessive weakness particularly in his legs—unable to stand. Ordered four rubbing-sheets, not wrung out, four times a day; head-baths three or four times a day; fever, notwithstanding, increased, and, patient was unable to bear the rubbing-sheet: upon which the treatment was changed to four packing-sheets, renewed every quarter of an hour, followed by a tepid bath for ten minutes. This process was repeated three times during the day.

Head became feverish. He took for this, a head-bath five minutes at a time. In a fortnight, fever left him completely; when only three packing-sheets a day, and cold bath after each, was ordered. In three weeks, patient was out of doors.

In the second week of his treatment, patient, besides several small eruptions, had five large boils, which opened in the first week, and discharged copiously for a fortnight, when his health improved daily; and before the expiration of the sixth week, he was perfectly well.

Remains of Fever strongly resembling Gout.—An artist caught a fever in Egypt. In Rome, his fingers and feet became enlarged, in appearance resembling gout, when he was treated for that complaint. Priessnitz at once declared this a mistake, and that it was the remains of the fever.

In three or four days after beginning the cure, patient had fever, and in ten days another strong attack: his feet and legs became much inflamed, attended with headache and great debility.

His former treatment was now abandoned for the following:

Three packing-sheets, one after the other, until warm; then the tepid bath for fifteen minutes: from that into the cold bath for two minutes, and return to the tepid again for fifteen or twenty minutes. This was to be repeated in the afternoon. When fever subsided, patient renewed his former treatment, and was perfectly cured in three months. I saw him in Rome the next year, when he was perfectly well; and as an act of gratitude to Mr. Priessnitz, he had caused to be painted a picture of the "eternal city," to send for his acceptance.

Intermittent Fever.—General R—— was attacked with intermittent fever at the siege of Mantua, in 1798. His complaint resisted all remedies: his liver became hardened and enlarged, exhibiting a tumour extending three fingers' breadth above his navel. Came to Gräfenberg thin as a skeleton, complexion nearly livid, unable to walk without the assistance of two persons. Obstinate indigestion and constipation; no motion for fifteen years, without aid;

congestion of blood to the head, and threatened apoplexy; insupportable sensitiveness to cold. Arrived at Gräfenberg in 1839; now restored to health: liver restored to normal size, with merely a slight swelling at epigastric region.

His treatment was:—morning, partial baths (tepid), twenty minutes, with strong friction; no water in the bath when patient first entered it, that being poured over his head and shoulders.

After one month of this treatment, sweating for half an hour, followed by partial bath for five minutes; noon, tepid sitz-bath (70 deg.) for half an hour; repeated in the afternoon.

In two months patient could walk alone. During the third month, sweating for an hour, and partial cold bath for five minutes; and sitz-baths were now cold; eighteen glasses of water, drunk daily; fourth month:—after sweating, the large plunge-bath, and friction by two men; twenty to twenty-four glasses of water, daily. Fifth month:—appetite good; commenced ascending the mountains. The douche found to excite too much: therefore abandoned.

August, 1840:—Left Gräfenberg: his liver softer, though not sensibly diminished. Recommended, whilst at home, to wear heating bandages always, and use cold ablutions, but not to transpire, unless pain of liver occurs.

In January, 1841, eruptions on the skin, and many ulcers, made their appearance.

August, 1841, returned to Gräfenberg, and commenced the same treatment as before: sweating one hour; plunge-bath and two partial baths a day; douche for five minutes every other day.

In November, had fever for twenty-five days, and pains in his hands, with open sores on his fingers for nine months; nails dropped off, and were replaced by new ones; fingers always wrapped in heating bandages. For the fever, six packing-sheets, changed every quarter of an hour, except the last: in this the patient remained longer, preparatory to a warm bath.

This was renewed twice a day.

Twenty-four glasses of water daily.

March, 1842.—Left Gräfenberg: liver reduced to one-half the size it was.

August, 1842.—Returned again to Gräfenberg, when his treatment was:—packing-sheet every morning one hour, followed by two rubbing-sheets; noon and afternoon, two rubbing-sheets.

October, 1842.—Was seen at his residence in health; pains from many old wounds no longer felt.

Patient aged forty-five. Ten years ago; caught cold, which ended in intermittent fever, which resisted the usual remedies; was cured at Gräfenberg as follows:—morning, packing-sheet and plunge-bath; noon, rubbing-sheet and sitz-bath; afternoon, as the morning.

Fever and ague returned every fourth day, when treatment was changed. Packing-sheet and tepid bath 62°, ten minutes; then into cold bath two minutes, and back again to tepid, with much friction; at noon, five rubbing-sheets; afternoon, as in the morning. The paroxysm over, resumed the former treatment until perfectly cured.

Fever and Ague.—S—— had fever, attended with ague; took nine packing and six rubbing-sheets, and three tepid baths; two of the tepid baths being followed by cold plunging bath. Cured the same day.

A lady attacked by slight fever and shivering, cured by five rubbing-sheets.

Sudden Fever.—Mrs. H——'s little boy awoke with fever; she kept him in a tepid bath, renewed with cold, until he trembled with cold; then put him to bed, where he immediately fell asleep, and awoke perfectly well. Priessnitz said the mother would have done as well, if she had given him a long sitz-bath.

Catarrh and Fever.—Child restless all night. Tepid bath (nearly cold) for a quarter of an hour; lean back in the bath so that the attendant may well rub the chest and throat. Afternoon, rubbing-sheet and tepid bath for a quarter of an hour.

After each bath, a head-bath for twelve minutes, each side of the head being alternately placed in the water. If this does not succeed, lay the back of the head in water, and well rub the forehead with wet hands. Rub the throat with wet hands three times a day. Eat no meat, and be much out of doors. Child, after first day's treatment, wretchedly cold; but pain in the head gone, and cough decreased.

Second day, pain in his legs, and weak; which Priessnitz said was the result of the fever. As the cough abated, treatment was moderated. Bath to be tepid. In the middle of the day, throat and chest to be rubbed. In the evening, a tepid bath eight minutes; head-bath as before; these were given in consequence of his feverish state in the night. If the body continued feverish, and the feet and legs cold at night, then heating bandages to the feet and legs, up to the fork, would have been applied all night.

Fever and Diarrhœa.—A Servant of my own, disturbed many times during the night with diarrhœa and fever, and with violent pain in his head and abdomen, was put into a packing-sheet for one hour and a quarter; a rubbing-sheet was then applied, followed by bandage round the waist; at noon, sitz-bath one hour and a quarter. This simple treatment effected a cure in a few hours.

Constipation and Fever.—Patient took tepid-bath, rubbed by three men for one hour and a half, getting out of the bath was dried and walked about the room every half-hour for ten minutes; followed by other treatment.

Second day, the above repeated twice, with the addition of packing-sheets and rubbing-sheets, in the interim.

General laxity of the bowels for several days, rest disturbed for two or three nights; could not rest the last night, diarrhœa and fever, strong pulse (110).

Morning, two packing-sheets, fifteen minutes each. In the first, patient felt (as he said) as though he was in boiling water; on the application of the second he felt cooler, after twenty-five minutes he was put into a cold bath and there remained until heat had left the arm-pits, which required seventeen minutes. Then a large towel was doubled four times and placed round his loins, drank six tumblers of water and went to bed.

At twelve o'clock all fever gone—to put an end to Diarrhœa, I ordered two rubbing sheets three minutes each, to be followed by tepid sitz-bath fifteen minutes, wet bandages and water to be drank as before.

At five o'clock sitz-bath twenty minutes.

Patient passed a good night, and next day found himself well.

P.S. I treated this case myself at Naples.

Cold Shivering by Day, and Feverish Heat when in Bed at Night.—A young man—ordered three rubbing-sheets on rising quite warm from bed in the morning; the same at noon, and in the afternoon drink plentifully of water.

Symptoms continuing—An additional three rubbing-sheets were used previous to going to bed, and when heat commenced in the night, the body bandage, which had been worn from the beginning was changed, and water drunk. If in a state of perspiration early in the morning, a tepid bath. This treatment had the desired effect.

XXXIX.—Congestion of the Lungs.

When the lungs are unsound sitz-baths are liable to cause a pain to be felt in that region, probably from causing congestion to them. I knew a case of this kind, and named it to Priessnitz who said, to have relieved this the patient should have been put into a very shallow tepid-bath, water two inches deep, and there rubbed by two men until the pain was removed.

In a case of Gout treated by an inexperienced person—where fears were entertained that congestion had taken place and castor oil was resorted to—he advised the same bath and friction, *until it* was removed.

A third case, where after being some time under the treatment a practitioner was embarrassed by his patient having fixed pain in his bowels, Priessnitz said, the bath applied with vigour for a considerable time would have been sure of removing it.

If a patient is ever lost in these cases, it is through the want of knowledge and the timidity of the practitioner.

XL.—Inflammations.

Inflammation of the Lungs.—This complaint originates in some obstruction, and is occasioned by an effort of nature to remove it. By bleeding the symptoms are reduced, but the cause remains, and consequently it frequently happens that under Hydropathic treatment inflammation returns, which then, by producing irritation on the surface, is extracted.

Mr. Priessnitz' married daughter, this year, returned to Gräfenberg, with her husband, to be cured of an epidemic which raged in Hungary. The husband was cured. The lady, with an eruption, went for two days into the country; on return the eruption had nearly subsided; it had gone to the lungs and inflammation resulted. She was put into tepid and cold baths thirty or forty times during the day. These positive means put an end to the inflammation in one day, and the next she was about as usual, quite well.

This apparently dangerous complaint, without any apparent cause, when taken quite in its infancy, is generally cured by the following simple means.

Place a cold packing-sheet several times doubled over the shoulders, chest, and back of the patient, whilst he takes a cold sitz-bath, for from half an hour to an hour, during the time use great friction to the feet and legs with hands dipped in water. All medical reasoning will be to the effect that this treatment must cause congestion to the lungs; but every day's practice at Gräfenberg proves the contrary.

Between the application of the above treatment, use a rubbing sheet.

If the head is affected, let the patient lay quiet in bed, with his head in a basin once or twice a day, from fifteen to thirty minutes, or much longer if necessary each time.

If fever, then resort to the tepid bath, until heat disappears under the arm-pits; this may require a long time, but must be persevered in.

The water of the bath must be continually renewed or it will become too warm.

I have known the sitz-bath, applied two or three times a day, completely cure an attack of this nature.

A lady, aged forty, attacked with inflammation of the lungs, was put into a tepid bath 62°, and kept there three hours and ten minutes, cold water being constantly poured over the shoulders, to bring down the temperature. Priessnitz frequently felt the chest and arm-pits; and in answer to patient's request to discontinue, he said if she did so until all parts were cool alike, her life would pay the forfeit.

After this, she took a cold bath twice a day, and wore the heating-bandage. In two months, she was perfectly cured. It should be remarked, that during the greater part of this times she felt a pain and hardness in the side, but this all subsided.

Spitting Blood and Inflammation.—A young man had inflammation of the lungs at Vienna, which ended in great debility and spitting of blood. Shortly after going to Gräfenberg he had another attack of inflammation of the lungs.

Treatment.—Tepid bath 62°, five minutes, then cold ten minutes, and back to the tepid ten minutes. This change from one bath to the other was repeated for nearly three hours, and ended about nine in the morning; at eleven o'clock, a sitz-bath fifteen minutes; afternoon, packing-sheet and cold bath for five minutes. Next day quite well of the attack; he continued packing-sheet and cold bath, morning and afternoon, and sitz-bath at noon; more heating-bandages on the chest. In ten weeks perfectly cured.

Inflammation in the Wind-pipe.—A lady—Chest, throat, and between the shoulders rubbed for five minutes with hands, and frequently dipped in cold water. During this time water was held in the mouth and changed when warm.

Bandages were applied to throat, shoulders, and waist.

Walked the same afternoon a short time.

Inflammation of the Brain.—Rubbing-sheets, head-baths, and bandages to the nape of the neck, back of the head, and some distance down the back, the rest of the body lightly covered. In an obstinate case, recourse must be had to a tepid bath 64° for a considerable time.

In all cases, whether in fever or not, where the head is attacked, large wet bandages may be applied, and changed every five minutes. Bandages to the whole of the head should not however be applied in general practice. The head ought to be free and the face washed often.

Inflammation of the Gums.—A child suffering indescribable pain, no sleep night or day.

One or two rubbing sheets, two or three times a day. Heating bandages to be applied to the head, as a turban, so that only the face can be seen, and changed every five or ten minutes. The same round the waist, from the hips to the arm-pits, and changed when warm.

If the body is confined, administer a cold water enema; if one is not sufficient, a second should be administered in half an hour; drink plentifully of water. Child out at play the third day.

XLI.—Gripes, Cholic, Diarrhœa, English Cholera, or Cholera Morbus.

All partake more or less of the same character; to describe the symptoms, nature, and medical treatment of these complaints, more volumes have been written than there are days in the year.

My object is not to inquire how such complaints arise, but to show how by the most simple and safe means they are to be cured.

Cholic.—This complaint invariably gives way to sitz-baths, clysters, bandages, and drinking plentifully of cold water.

A patient suffering from pain in the bowels for some days, was ordered injections three times a day, notwithstanding the bowels were perfectly free.

W——, taken with sickness and griping pains, could retain nothing on his stomach, supposed that it arose from eating unripe fruit. An injection of cold water was first resorted to; one not being sufficient, a second in half an hour was administered, and during the day ten others. Then two rubbing sheets, followed by a tepid bath, with great friction, and large bandage, three hours afterwards, a sitz-bath, tepid, fifteen minutes.

Again, after a lapse of three hours, the former process. This put an end to the gripes the same day.

An Austrian officer, attacked with violent pain in the abdomen, which extended through to the back. Great heat and pain in the head, with cold feet.

Priessnitz wetted the body all over with cold water, particularly the feet, and without drying the parts thus wetted, ordered the patient to sit quite naked near to the window, which was open, for one hour in a sitz-bath, his servant rubbing him the whole time. Patient was then covered up well in bed to bring on re-action, the pains of which for a short time were worse than cholic. The attack was put an end to by this one application, or it was to have been renewed in the morning.

The singular part of this treatment is, that the body was thus exposed to the inclemency of a Siberian winter, wet and naked, for one hour. When asked why he adopted such positive treatment, Priessnitz said, because there was a great tendency to intestinal inflammation. The patient was out and well next day.

Dysentery and Diarrhœa.—For the information of the general reader, it may be well to state, that Dysentery is brought on by damp, cold, or unripe fruit, and is attended by the evacuation of bloody glaires, violent pain of the stomach, burning at the arms, and spasms of the bladder, a constant desire to evacuate without being able to render anything but glaires. Diarrhœa is attended with many of these symptoms, but there is no blood in the evacuation. Hereafter it will be shewn how both these complaints are to be treated.

Cold clysters, rubbing-sheets, sitz-baths, and bandage, are the chief agents in the cure of these complaints. When attended with inflammation take three or four sitz-baths a day, and change the body bandages every ten minutes.

In Diarrhœa or Dysentery the patient should take but little exercise.

When Diarrhœa is recent, it is sufficient to drink plentifully of water, wear a bandage round the wrist, eat little, and that of farinaceous food.

Diarrhœa is often the work of nature to carry off prejudicial humours; which ought not to be prevented. At the same time it must not be suffered to continue too long without resorting to measures to check it. A patient came to Gräfenberg who had suffered six weeks from this complaint, which had reduced him almost to a skeleton. He was cured in a few days.

Where abundant evacuations of glaires are alternate with constipation, cold injections are a great relief. If patients in Cholera, Diarrhœa, Cholic, or Dysentery, cannot sleep, administer a very cold foot-bath, water only half an inch deep, for fifteen minutes. Let the feet, legs, and thighs be rubbed with wet hands the whole time, then the patient should walk bare-footed in the chamber for ten minutes.

Dysentery.—Begin with one or two rubbing-sheets, then cold injections every quarter of an hour for two or three hours.

Then tepid sitz-bath, rather warmer than usual, for half an hour, followed by a large heating bandage doubled three or four times, from before the hips to the arm-pits, leaving the arms free. Change this every ten or fifteen minutes. Let the covering to the bed be light, but keep the feet warm. Drink large quantities of cold water.

When the bandage has been changed three or four times, if the patient is better, let him remain quiet; otherwise repeat the treatment.

Miss B——, attacked with dysentery attended with great pain; ordered four sitz-baths in a day, one hour each large bandage from hips to arm-pits; changed often.

Took them two days, and one in the night. These chilled her exceedingly, which Priessnitz said was as it ought to be.

Diarrhœa.—A delicate lady, ordered not to drink milk for some days, but sixteen to twenty glasses of water; take but little exercise; at noon wash with cold water; at eleven o'clock, cold sitz-bath, twenty minutes, then walk a few times in the room, with only dry sheet over the person; then sitz-bath again for twenty minutes; repeat this a third time to complete the hour.

F——, had diarrhœa two days, when Priessnitz said, "If you are not in pain, do nothing; if the contrary, take a morning rubbing-sheet, and sitz-bath three quarters of an hour; noon, the same; afternoon, sitz-bath three quarters of an hour; change bandages and walk less; drink plentifully of water."

A—— had Diarrhœa whilst travelling, as he could not procure sitz-bath, he lay in bed, changed bandages every half hour, and drank freely of water. This treatment sufficed.

Chronic Diarrhœa.—Morning, packing-sheet from hips to arm-pits until warm, then cold bath; noon, two rubbing-sheets and sitz-bath half-an-hour; evening, sitz-bath half-an-hour; or in the morning, sitz-bath for half an hour, then walk, return and take cold bath; drink plentifully of water and wear large bandages.

Pain in the Bowels.—Tepid sitz-bath 62° for three quarters of an hour; rubbing the abdomen all the time; in a simple case this puts an end to the pain at once.

Severe Pain in the Bowels.—Tepid sitz-bath, half an hour to an hour; much rubbing with wet hands on the back, stomach, and abdomen when in the bath; no exertion of mind or body; eat only of one thing; drink much water. When constipated, or had pain in the bowels, extended the period of the sitz bath. Patient's recovery quite marvellous.

The sitz-bath may be resorted to two or three times a day, and also rubbing-sheet, if the case proves obstinate.

Pain in Bowels and Diarrhœa.—Ordered sitz-bath fifteen minutes, walk gently about the room five minutes, then repeat the sitz-bath fifteen minutes, and again walk for five minutes, and after third time take sitz-bath. Put on a large bandage well wrung out, and change it every quarter of an hour. If not cured in three or four hours, repeat the above treatment. If obstinate use cold injections.

Relaxed Bowels.—Three rubbing-sheets and a sitz-bath on rising from bed, for ten minutes in the morning; one rubbing sheet, and sitz-bath twenty minutes at noon; the same repeated in the afternoon. If not better, a clyster of cold water on going to bed; bandage, and drink water as usual.

A young lady, troubled with relaxed bowels for some days—

Morning, three rubbing-sheets, and immediately after, tepid bath for fifteen minutes; large bandage; at two o'clock two rubbing sheets.

These simple means effected a cure; if they had not, the sitz-bath was to have been resorted to again.

English Cholera.—A Russian General attacked with English Cholera, was suffering extreme torture when Priessnitz came. He ordered three rubbing-sheets, five minutes interim between each; patient then to be put to bed for half-an-hour, and well covered up to promote heat; this was followed by a cold sitz-bath of 30 or 40 minutes; drank plentifully of water and wore a large heating bandage.

This one application effected a complete cure; had it not, the General was to have repeated the treatment in the afternoon.

XLII.—Consumption.

Mr. Priessnitz thinks that in the great majority of cases consumption is curable until the age of fourteen or fifteen, when the complaint generally assumes a more serious aspect.

Young people are often considered consumptive when they really are not so. A young lady of my acquaintance, having all the symptoms, was ordered to Italy, where, notwithstanding the climate, the malady seemed to increase. She went to Gräfenberg, when Mr. Priessnitz at once declared it was not consumption, that it was a contraction of the chest. Two months' treatment caused the chest to expand and restored the patient to robust health. Dr. Johnson says, "One thing of which I am convinced is, that the true principle of treating consumption is to support the patient's strength to the utmost;" and it must be remembered that the great aim and principal effect of the Water-cure is to *strengthen the system*, thereby giving the inherent curative power the fairest opportunity of doing its own work.

It must however be observed, that when consumption has fairly set in, neither water or drugs will arrest its progress. A friend of mine writes me most sensibly on this subject: "I fully believe," says he, "if all girls were to *wash thoroughly every* day, more than three-fourths who now go into consumption would be saved."

XLIII.—Cramps.

Rubbing-sheets, and rubbing powerfully with wet hands, for a considerable time, particularly the feet, are efficient means of cure; after each application let the patient remain quiet. If the hands or feet become cold, apply friction again to them and the parts affected.

Mr. Brown finding patient nearly dead from Cramp, immediately administered an enema, then a rubbing-sheet with great friction, followed by a tepid bath for nearly an hour, the enema took effect whilst under the friction, rubbing-sheets and baths were repeated three times before mid-day with good effect.

In the afternoon, rubbing-sheets were used, and friction with wet hands.

Cramp-Cough.—I knew a case of this nature which was most successfully treated at Gräfenberg.

Morning, two or three packing-sheets followed by tepid bath; noon, tepid sitz-bath, quarter of an hour; afternoon, morning treatment renewed.

The Crisis was attended with inflammation and ulcers of the throat.

Tepid-baths, were administered twice a day, for ten to fifteen minutes, changing alternately from hot to cold and back to hot. To subdue fever which was very active in the night, the patient took a plunge or two into a cold bath before going to bed.

Bandage on Chest at night, in addition to that round the loins.

Cramps in the Stomach.—Patient's complaint was cramp in the stomach, weak digestion, great nervous sensibility. Packing-sheet one hour, and tepid-bath in the morning, four minutes, with great friction; then three successive plunges into tepid, cold, and tepid-bath, to remain in the last four minutes; noon, rubbing-sheet five minutes, followed by sitz-bath ten minutes; afternoon, repeat morning treatment, wear bandage day and night, and drink twelve tumblers of water daily.

In a short time, the tepid-bath was relinquished for the cold-bath; and the douche was used for two minutes, as a longer period was found to disagree with the patient. A diarrhœa was cured by the addition of sitz-baths; at which time the douche was not persevered in.

XLIV.—Asthma.

I was astonished at the wonderful effects of the Water-cure treatment, in cases of Asthma. One night, Priessnitz was called up to a patient under the cure, who was almost suffocated.

A tepid sitz-bath for thirty minutes with great friction of the abdomen completely relieved him. This patient was perfectly cured in three months.

A patient whose age was thirty-five suffered from chest complaint, asthma, torpid circulation, and stricture. For some time three rubbing-sheets a day only were prescribed, then a tepid sitz-bath; and when he evidenced the cure of the Asthma, by ascending with ease the highest mountains, the general treatment was resorted to.

In three months the stricture was quite cured. Left Gräfenberg the fourth month.

The following interesting case, came under my especial notice.

Mr. M——, aged 26, afflicted with Asthma for three years, tried all the baths in Germany, and then determined on going to Gräfenberg: *en route*, he was confined to an hotel for eight days. When he arrived, which was on the 4th January, 1846, he could with difficulty walk a quarter of a mile.

Inclement as the weather was, Priessnitz, at once ordered him into a tepid bath, and stripped him of all flannels; next day he began the following treatment, until warm.

Morning, packing-sheet, tepid-bath; noon, rubbing-sheet, and tepid sitz-bath; afternoon, the same. In a short time tepid water was discontinued for cold.

In about three weeks, two large boils appeared and broke, when he was so much better, as to ascend the highest mountains, his health improved so fast, that, first in the morning, he was seen up to his middle in snow, always without hat, neckcloth or great coat.

He was cured in about four months.

XLV.—Surgical Operations, Accidents, etc.

Amputation.—The Surgeon's profession would be a very poor one if Hydropathy were generally understood.

If a finger, hand, or foot, be nearly severed from the body, they should be put into the best possible form, bandaged, and placed between two pieces of wood; over this a large bandage: the former may be wetted often without being removed.

A friend of mine in Italy had the misfortune, whilst botanising, to fall from one rock to another, where he hung by his foot. This caused a compound fracture, and the loss of his foot. I asked Mr. Priessnitz what ought to have been done,—he said his shepherd would have known better than to have cut off the foot; a stiff one being preferable to none at all. The foot should have been healed as above described, a large bandage applied from the toes up to the top of the thighs constantly wetted; this would have kept the limb cold. As fever or inflammation must proceed from the part afflicted, it is evident if the heat is extracted thence, neither can ensue. The splinters would have come away of themselves, and the patient might have been spared the loss of his foot, and several months of severe suffering and loss of health.

Crushed Finger.—A farmer at Gräfenberg had his finger smashed by a large stone rolling against it; so that it hung by the skin. It was put together, bandaged, and so fixed between two pieces of wood; over this a larger bandage was placed, the under part kept constantly wet. When pain ensued, the elbow was put into cold water for twenty minutes. The finger, though stiffer than the others, was preserved.

Fainting Fit.—Open the window to admit fresh air; unfasten the dress. Sprinkle water on the face and put the feet into a foot pan, with water only up to the instep, and let the attendant rub feet and legs up to the knees.

Effects of Falls.—A young man who came with nervous fever, one day, whilst labouring under violent palpitation, to which he was subject, fell, and so hurt the back of his head, as to be insensible for half an hour. Priessnitz, being sent for, ordered a foot-bath and rubbing with wet hands up to the knee. Opened his waistcoat, rubbed the chest, and threw cold water into his face. The friction and foot-bath continued for an hour, when patient was ordered a sitz-bath for thirty minutes. Bandages to waist and head.

Another party fell and injured his large toe against a stone. Ordered three cold foot-baths a day, fifteen minutes each time, and bandage to be kept continually wet.

Count C. fell down stairs, and afterwards felt pain in his side. Bandaged the part. Next day a tepid bath for one hour. As the Count was not young, this was not persevered in. Sitz-baths were substituted.

A. fell from his horse and injured his elbow and arm.

Arm and elbow placed in a tepid bath for an hour.

Repeated three times a day. Arm bandaged night and day.

Bruised Shin.—Three sitz-baths a day 60°; bandage the leg from ancle to above the knee, and keep it raised. Throw tepid water over foot and leg several times a day.

Foot-baths may be resorted to, if the patient is already under hydropathic treatment: otherwise not, as they draw bad matter downwards, and might prevent the wound from healing.

B. trod upon a nail which entered his foot. His foot was put for an hour twice or thrice a day into tepid water, and he wore a bandage on the part.

In all cases of the kind—either by cutting with sharp instruments or otherwise, put the wounded part into tepid water until it ceases bleeding, then bandage it, and afterwards use cold baths several times a day to the part.

Bandages must extend both ways beyond the wound, to carry off the inflammation from the part. Viz.—If the calf of the leg be wounded, the bandage ought to begin at the ancle, and be continued up to the knee. In all cases take one or two tepid sitz-baths a day. They prevent the head being affected.

Tape Worms.—Rubbing-sheets once or twice a day, bandage always round the waist, cold injections morning and evening, and drink plentifully of water.

For other worms recourse must be had to the general treatment.

Sea Sickness.—Wear a large thick bandage on chest and abdomen; and if it does not prevent, it will mitigate sea-sickness.

Apoplexy and Paralysis.—Instantly put patient into tepid-bath, water about two inches deep, throw cold water over head and shoulders, and use immense friction with wet hands for a very long time. For a wonderful case of cure of Apoplexy, refer to the letter written from Gräfenberg to the New York Tribune.

Lock Jaw.—The same as for Apoplexy.

A Belgian Doctor had a paralytic stroke two months previous to coming to Gräfenberg. In a fortnight he had another; when he could neither speak nor eat, and was too feeble to take the bath.

Sixteen rubbing-sheets a day, four at a time, restored him the use of his faculties in two days.

A crochet-needle was, by accident, driven into the side of a young lady; a surgeon lanced the part and extracted it, when Priessnitz simply ordered a bandage to the part, to be changed every quarter of an hour until inflammation subsided, and subsequently, as often as it became dry. After the first day no inconvenience was felt. A green matter exuded from the wound, which P. said was nothing more than usual in such circumstances.

Scalds.—Put the part affected into cold water, or apply a cold affusion for an hour two or three times a day. Wear a bandage continually wet; when the inflammation has subsided, put a dry bandage over the wet one.

Burns.—If a burn be bad, and the patient cannot endure the application of water, in that case use tow or lint; but if possible, wring a bandage well out, apply it to the burn, and put a dry one over it. Change the bandage often; but if this is too painful, let it remain, and wet it often. A cold bath applied as a derivative will afford great relief; *i. e.* if the leg is burnt take a foot-bath; if the hand, put the elbow in cold water, &c.

Rupture of the Tendon Achilles.—A friend of mine, running across the road, heard the crack of a whip; and supposed at first that some one had struck his leg with a whip, but he soon found he could not put his foot to the ground, that he had met with an accident called *coup de fouet,* or a rupture of the tendon Achilles in the calf of his leg. The only treatment for this, which effected an immediate cure, was binding it up in a surgeon's bandage very tight, and keeping that wet night and day.

Accidents to the Head.—A man chopping wood struck a child a back blow on the forehead; the wound was wetted with tepid water for some time, and then a bandage was applied.

Two tepid sitz-baths were administered during the day.

Another child seven years old, fell against a stone and laid his forehead open.

Bandage applied, and wetted occasionally without being taken off; a dry one kept over it.

Another bandage at the back of the neck, renewed often.

Tepid sitz-bath fifteen minutes, three times a day. Feverish symptoms arose during the night; sitz-bath renewed.

Prince Ruspoli, Lord Anson, and another were galloping along a road at the dusk of the evening, not perceiving a drain, two of their horses fell into it. Two of the party were taken up insensible. On being brought into Freywalden, they were instantly put into tepid baths of 65°.

The prince having fallen on his temple was much stunned; four men rubbed him in the bath, in five minutes he became conscious and assisted in rubbing himself; in ten minutes he felt cold. After being in the bath twenty-five minutes he was taken out, well dried and put to bed, with bandages on his head and back of the neck, and but slight covering. After an hour's repose, a tepid sitz-bath was administered for an hour. During the night patient suffered great pain in his head. Next day he was out of doors, but took three sitz-baths during the day; in the morning for an hour; the others, half an hour each time. Bandages always to the injured part. In a few days he was quite well.

The prince's friend was threatened with congestion in the head, and had great pain in the stomach; the fæces were nearly black. He took many injections; three sitz-baths daily, an hour and a half each time, and one during the night. This treatment effected his cure.

Cuts and Wounds.—For a clean cut, it will often be sufficient to close the wound at once, and cover it with a dry bandage, so as to exclude the air.

A bruise, or jagged cut, should be bound up, and covered with a wet bandage; and this, when inflammation has subsided, must be covered with a dry one. Do not remove the under bandage, but pour water on it occasionally, and cover it again with the dry one. Let the bandage extend both ways beyond the wound, to conduct away the heat from it.

Calf of Leg torn off.—Dr. Scontetton, surgeon to the forces at Strasburg, states, "A soldier trying to descend at night from the walls of the barracks, fell, and tore the flesh off the calf of his leg. The doctor put the lacerated flesh together as well as he could, and bound the leg and thigh up in a bandage; a trough was then made in a slanting position in which he placed the leg. Over the man's head he fixed a cask of water with a tube, from which the man was to keep the bandage constantly wet.[6] By this treatment alone a cure was effected in a fortnight, during which time the man suffered no pain, nor was even deprived of his appetite."

Sprained Shoulder.—A patient fell down an ice-berg and severely bruised his shoulder, so that he could not raise his hand. The bruise was immediately saturated with cold water for an hour, and cold wet cloths applied for a long time. When inflammation had subsided, a heating bandage was applied and renewed when dry. Elbow bath twice a day, fifteen minutes each.

This treatment was repeated two or three times a day.

Accident to the Eye.—A child five years old, ran a knife into the ball of the eye. Cold wet bandages perfected a cure. The blue of the eye ran, but the boy, now fifteen years of age, sees perfectly well.

Swelling of a Vein—Varicose Veins.—A young lady was afflicted with swelled vein just over the large toes of both feet; the swelling in one foot shortly disappeared, the other became more developed, the foot and ancle inflamed.

I wrote to Priessnitz, who advised "a cold foot-bath, three times a day, for twenty minutes; water up to the ancle and not to be changed. After the bath, rub the foot (omitting the affected part) and leg, particularly in front, up to the knee, until heat is restored; then apply a bandage (well wrung out) to the foot and leg up to the knee, always changing before dry. If an eruption or swelling take place on the foot, take a sitz-bath half an hour, twice a day, and the sweating process, followed by cold bath every other day. Do not perspire more than an hour. The foot should be kept a little elevated."

Patient not getting better, and the medical men declaring the case, in their opinion, incurable, she went to Gräfenberg. The following is the treatment pursued there:—Packing-sheets for fifteen minutes; changed for another of twenty minutes; and cold plunge-bath morning and evening; between which douched twice a day, and a sitz-bath taken; always wearing foot and leg and waist bandage.

Priessnitz, on seeing the case, declared the complaint was not a local one, that "it was a general derangement of the nervous system", and so it turned out, as veins in the arms, thighs, and elsewhere enlarged and diminished under the treatment. Both feet and legs now became swollen and inflamed up to the knee, so that patient was obliged to move on crutches. Treatment increased. Length of cold bath and douche extended to five minutes each. To prevent the pain that must have attended the limbs, in so inflamed a state, coming in contact with water, the bandages remained on those parts whilst taking those baths. This crisis continued for two months, when it began to recede, then came again in a more moderate form; receded and again made its appearance a third and last time. Catamenia became regular, appetite good, and patient could walk without assistance. The cure was effected in ten months. It is now upwards of two years since the party left Gräfenberg, and she is perfectly well.

By this it will be seen, that that which is produced by the treatment, must be made to recede under the treatment. Had Priessnitz relinquished any part of it at the most trying moment, the cure would not have been effected.

Speaking to him of varicose or enlarged veins, he said "they are generally curable. I had a patient with an enlarged vein in his foot, when on the ground the vein became full, measuring nearly two inches; this was cured in eighteen months."

Sprains.—In all cases of sprains, rub the part, with hands dipped in water, for a long time; the oftener the better, and put on a wet bandage, which when heat has subsided, change for a heating bandage.

If the sprain is a bad one, apply a cold bath or cold affusion to the part for half an hour, then the wet, and afterwards the heating bandage, which change often.

The bath should be repeated thrice a day, and friction used the whole time.

If general treatment is necessary, then packing-sheets. Tepid bath and tepid sitting baths must be resorted to.

Sprained Ankle.—Put the foot immediately into cold water, and rub foot, ankle, and leg up to the knee for an hour, particularly the wounded part. The water of the bath, after the first time, only up to the instep, but repeated three or four times a day. Bandage the foot, ankle, and leg up to the knee; first, with quite wet bandages, and when inflammation has somewhat subsided, then with heating bandage. The foot should not be allowed to remain quiet. If not able to move about, the patient should put a rolling pin under his foot and keep that in movement. By these means a sprained ankle is cured in a few days, that without it might continue for a month or longer.

Wound in the Abdomen.—A lad leaning upon a piece of wood, hurt his abdomen; it was rubbed with cold water for half an hour, followed by sitz-bath half an hour twice a day.

Bleeding at the Nose.—Sprinkle the face with water, bandage the back of the neck and the loins; shallow foot bath, where obstinate. Bandage the genitals and change the bandage often.

Dr. Gibbs states, that whilst at Gräfenberg, he was greatly troubled with bleeding at the nose. He tried bandages at the back of the neck and foot-bath to no purpose. Priessnitz then ordered him two packing-sheets in succession, the first fifteen minutes, the other twenty-five minutes, followed by cold bath. This treatment had the desired effect.

I knew a case where a man bled profusely at the nose. He put his feet up to the calves of his legs in cold water, and the bleeding stopped in ten minutes.

A child had a blow on the nose, which occasioned it to bleed frequently.

Bandage worn on the forehead for a week or two, and foot baths, completed a cure.

Spitting Blood, Sickness, etc.—This is sometimes occasioned by piles. Sitz-baths (tepid 62°) may be taken; bandages worn on the waist always, and on the chest at night. All irritation should be avoided, and repose of body and mind observed. Water ought to be drunk abundantly. Bleeding of the lungs, the effect of pulmonary consumption, is not curable. To distinguish the difference between cases requires the experience of such a genius as Priessnitz.

XLVI.—Small Pox, Measles, Hooping Cough, Croup, Scarlatina, Colds, Shivering, etc.

All these complaints form the easiest and surest part of Priessnitz's practice. No child or adult ever died at Gräfenberg of any of them. This fact, attested as it is by all writers on Hydropathy, leads one to look on the incertitude of medical practice in diseases incidental to children, with wonder and dismay.

Priessnitz considers these complaints wholesome, being the medium chosen by Nature for relieving the system.

On their appearance, his great aim is to strengthen the patient, and eliminate the morbific matters by the pores of the skin. It is frequently asked, "But does not the hydropathic process drive the virus into the system?" No, on the contrary, the packing-sheet acts as a poultice to the whole body; and this, followed by a tepid bath, causes an outward action, and the system is cooled and relieved through miles of drainage (the pores), the true medium through which relief can with certainty be obtained.

A young man with measles, at Gräfenberg, had as many as 400 packing-sheets applied in about fourteen days.

Small-Pox.—Small-pox, of all diseases, is that which should be treated hydropathically; because by its operation the morbid matters are thrown out by the pores of the skin, upon which it rarely leaves any of those scars so detrimental to the beauty of the person.

In the Water-cure, judiciously treated, the small-pox is under no circumstances attended with danger, nor is the patient reduced in strength as under any other treatment. "Small pox," Priessnitz says, "instead of being suppressed, ought to be encouraged, as it relieves the system of humours that ought to be carried out of it, and is a healthy process." At one period the profession were as much at fault in the treatment of small-pox, as they now are in that of cholera. No means were left untried, but they failed in arresting its ravages. Jenner's discovery was hailed as an intervention of Providence, and he was voted two grants in parliament. If Priessnitz is right, this discovery may be hailed as a curse rather than a blessing. He states that the insertion of poisonous matter into the blood of a healthy subject produces poisonous consequences, is repugnant to our feelings, and at variance with the laws of nature.

In small pox, where there is much eruption on the face, a muslin handkerchief, wetted, may be used as a bandage to the part.

If the head is much affected, head-bath and wet bandages must be resorted to.

Bandage the back and thighs if they require it. In these complaints, as in all others, if the bowels require opening, use injections. Drink plentifully of water.

I treated a young lady in small-pox as follows:—

First day—patient was confined to the sofa with head-ache and general lassitude; next morning, fever and several pustules: two packing-sheets, the first twenty minutes, the other twenty-five minutes; and tepid bath 70° for eight minutes. Afternoon—As the packing-sheet did not heat so soon as that in the morning, it was not changed, but patient remained in it an hour and a quarter—the tepid bath eight minutes—drank sixteen tumblers of water, windows always open. Second day, eruption much increased over the body and face; treatment as before. Third and fourth day, eruption increased; same treatment persevered in. Fifth day, treatment only in the morning. Sixth day, eruption decreasing. Eighth day, catamenia, all treatment suspended; which it should be observed would not have been the case had any fever remained. Tenth day, patient out walking, eruption nearly gone. Twelfth and thirteenth day, one rubbing-sheet on getting out of bed. It should be stated, that the wet bandage was *perpetually* worn during the treatment.

Patient quite as well and as strong as before the attack. Complexion much clearer.

The most extraordinary thing to be observed is, that the patient was not confined to bed for an hour—felt no disposition to scratch herself. The tongue, after third day, was perfectly clean, and her rest after the first night undisturbed.

The fever was taken out the first day, from which time she was not inconvenienced in the least. This young lady had been twice vaccinated.

The second and third day a smell remained in the room after patient was taken out of the sheet and bath, that was perfectly intolerable; which shows that the virus was taken out, and accounts for the eruption being so mild.

Another friend of mine, 46 years of age, caught the small pox, though he had been vaccinated twice. He was treated much in the same way, and was out of doors quite well the twelfth day, never having been confined to his bed for an hour. Windows open night and day.

In all eruptive complaints, packing-sheets allay the fever. To effect this, where the fever is strong, they should be changed once or twice, or even oftener. When there is much eruption, the heat of the bath which follows the wet sheet must be increased in extraordinary cases even to 80 deg.

The packing-sheet process and the tepid bath must be used twice a-day; patient must drink abundance of water; windows of the room ought to be always open; if constipated, clysters; waist bandages in all cases.

This treatment persevered in, must cure all eruptive and other fevers. No fear need exist as to the eruption by these means being driven in—all experience shows it is the way to bring it to the surface.

Dr. Farr declares himself a convert to the Water-cure in cases of eruption and other fevers, and did me the favour of writing the following letter:—

"Miss —— for two days had a sensation of languor, drowsiness, and pain in the head and loins, with sickness and fever. On the third day there appeared on the face small red spots, and successively on the inferior parts, until the fifth day! these rose into pimples, and then filled with puriform matter; dry hard scales formed, and on these falling off, pits or marks were left on some of them. The cold water cure had been commenced when I first saw her, which had cut the fever, and altered the character of the eruption; but as soon as the pustules began to form, the nature of the disease was no longer a matter of doubt; the pustules were as well developed, and went through their regular changes as well and as perfectly as though no application of cold had been made use of. This was the first case of small-pox I saw this winter at Nice, but shortly after several others occurred, and some of them of the confluent kind. I must confess I was surprised at the complete success of the cold water cure in this case.

"W. FARR."

"Nice, 13th April, 1848.["]

Scarlatina and Measles.—These two complaints are treated alike:—

Morning, packing-sheet twenty-five minutes, then change it for another for twenty-five minutes, followed by tepid bath 64° for ten minutes. Bandages. If the eruption is extensive, heat of the bath must be increased.

Repeat the treatment in the afternoon. If there is much heat between the hours of treatment, take as many rubbing-sheets one after the other as are necessary to subdue it. Much water should be drunk.

Scarlatina.—This complaint, on its first indication, is often subdued by the following simple means:—

Two or three packing-sheets. Large bandage round the waist. Drink water and walk out. A few hours afterwards repeat the same.

If obstinate, two or three packing-sheets, changed when warm, followed by tepid bath 64°.

If in scarlatina, or measles, the throat is affected, drink often in small quantities. Renew the packing-sheet frequently. When fever is diminished, slight perspiration in packing-sheet for half an hour; then tepid bath twenty minutes, with friction. Bread and milk diet.

A child, eleven years old, exhibited symptoms of scarlatina. Dry and hot all over the body. Stitch from chest to back. Was put into a tepid bath 64° and rubbed for an hour, cold water being continually thrown over its shoulders; child extremely cold; walked out. The same operation performed again in the afternoon and twice the next day put an end to the attack.

Hooping Cough.—Rub the child well all over, particularly the chest and back of the neck with hands continually dipped in cold water; or use a rubbing sheet. Bandage the chest, breast, and loins. If sufficiently strong, let the child lie in bed until quite hot, then tepid bath 64° and use great friction until quite chilled. If fever be present, a packing-sheet should precede the tepid bath, and afterwards a bandage round the waist.

Hooping cough may also be treated thus:—

Tepid bath, with great friction, for ten minutes in the morning; two rubbing-sheets at mid-day; the same in the afternoon: head-bath before going to bed; chest and body bandaged and changed often; drink much water.

Mumps.—Begin with rubbing-sheets; then packing-sheets and tepid-bath.

Bandage the throat, loins, and side of the head affected.

Change the bandages often, keep the mouth full of water, and change it when warm.

Croup with Sore Throat and Cough.—A child, on awaking in the morning, had face very red and found much difficulty in breathing. Treatment:—

A cold water injection, then two rubbing-sheets, and bandage all round the body from the throat to the hips.

An enema did not act, but appeared to cool the body; it remained in the body eight minutes. When discharged, another rubbing-sheet and wet bandage were applied. Breathing free, and child slept until morning. Then well rubbed in bath 62° for ten minutes.

Ate little breakfast. Dined on rice pudding.

Afternoon. Flushed and feverish.

Priessnitz, who now saw the patient, approved of what had been done, and said if the croup had continued, eight or ten rubbing-sheets ought to have been administered; allowing ten to twenty minutes between each; depending upon the violence of attack and strength of patient.

Evening. Patient was feverish, when the following was ordered:—

Body, *but not* the feet, to be enveloped in packing-sheet, and there remain until feet were warm: then tepid-bath 64° ten minutes. If the feet are cold in the bath, rub them with wet hands until a good circulation is produced.

In the night, fever abated and the child slept soundly.

Next day croup nearly gone and appetite good.

Another child with croup was treated in the same way on the first day. At nine o'clock at night, chest, windpipe, and between the shoulders, were rubbed for some time with wet hands; then the waist, throat, and chest were bandaged.

Slept well, but flushed and feverish in the morning; complained of sore throat. Packing-sheet until hot, and tepid-bath 64°.

Still feverish.

At noon, rubbing-sheet, not wrung out. If no fever and appetite, to go out.

Repeat rubbing-sheet in the afternoon.

Should fever continue, packing-sheet followed by rubbing-sheets. This was not necessary.

Second day. Tepid bath in the morning, and rubbing-sheets at twelve and five o'clock. Both children cured in three days.

A child seven years old, subject all his life to severe attacks of croup, on being seized with one at Gräfenberg, was treated as follows:—

Rubbed between the shoulders, and on the chest, for some minutes with wet hands; then lifted out of bed, and well rubbed all over, especially in the legs, in a very wet sheet from five to eight minutes.

A wet handkerchief was then put on as a shawl, and a bandage round the waist; when the patient was allowed to return to bed for ten minutes; after which the same treatment was repeated. This induced sleep, and he awoke free from all signs of croup.

At twelve o'clock there was a relapse, when the rubbing was renewed, and bandage applied to the waist.

At five o'clock in the afternoon, tepid-bath 64° for some minutes, and patient slept all night in bandage and wet shawl.

The treatment was renewed second day.

A child three years old, also liable to attacks of croup, on being attacked one evening about nine o'clock, was instantly rubbed on the chest, windpipe, and between the shoulders, followed by a general rubbing in rubbing-sheet for five minutes; then bandages were applied to throat, chest, and round the waist.

This apparently gave great relief, but in the morning he awoke flushed and feverish, complaining of his throat. A rubbing-sheet followed by a tepid-bath for some minutes, was resorted to; and at twelve o'clock another rubbing-sheet followed. Fever having subsided, he was allowed to go out.

At five o'clock the rubbing-sheet was repeated. He wore the bandage on his throat down to his chest day and night, changing it when dry. Had fever continued, he was to have lain in packing-sheet at five o'clock until warm, instead of the rubbing-sheet. Since this time both children have been perfectly well.—*August, 1845.*

Ophthalmia.—Inflammation of the eyes is generally catarrhal or rheumatic, and requires the same treatment as rheumatism and gout. I never saw it acute, but always chronic.

To the rheumatic treatment, Priessnitz adds eye-baths, and the douche. The latter must be received in the joined hands; from which, water coming from a height will rebound as high as the eyes. Head-baths are equally indispensable, as well as fomentations, to these organs. Chronic ophthalmia, even at Gräfenberg, is most obstinate, and requires a long course of treatment.

A captain thus attacked, felt, after several head-baths which he continued for three quarters of an hour, a pungent pain in the head, accompanied by swelling of the ears. An abscess was expected in one of these organs, when the pain gave way to a virulent deposit, formed in the thick part of the cheek; after this, the eyes were re-established.

Another sufferer came to Gräfenberg, with an exfoliation in the corner of the eye. To the whole of the treatment, Priessnitz added eye-baths; after each of which, the invalid was to look fixedly at the light, and immediately re-plunge the eyes into cold water. This man, who was perfectly blind on coming, was, on leaving Gräfenberg, able to read with spectacles.

A third patient presented a very remarkable case of blindness, the result of a cold caught during hunting, by which he lost his sight. He had been nine months blind, when he arrived at Gräfenberg; after each process of perspiration, which he submitted to twice a day, the bath and the head-bath, matter mixed with blood came from the eyes. One might say that some pounds exuded from the eyes in the course of three weeks. I did not see the termination of this cure, before leaving Gräfenberg; but I can affirm, that the last time I spoke to the invalid, he could distinguish colours, and also objects at a certain distance.

Itch and Ringworm.—These diseases are more easily cured by cold water, than by any other means. The process of perspiration in the wet sheet, leads to success; but ringworm is frequently more difficult to cure than the itch. It requires longer time, and a more energetic use of cold water.—The douche is also indispensable in cases of ringworm, in order to bring the morbid humours to the skin. The most difficult ringworms to cure, are those which have been driven in by bad treatment. This disease is really equal to the gout, in point of obstinacy, for it re-appears upon the skin after the use of the douche a long time. After the process of perspiration, and cold baths too, it again shows itself under forms much more serious in their aspect, than in the beginning.

Cold, Cough, with Inflammation.—A lady was ordered—

Packing-sheet, half or three quarters of an hour, then tepid bath 64° for an hour, twice a day. After first day much better. Third day cured. If patient is fatigued by staying in bath so long, let him come out and walk about the room for a few minutes, then enter the bath again.

Major——, a strong man, pursued the following treatment and was cured the third day.

Morning—Packing-sheet, two and a half hours, and tepid bath 64°, ten minutes. Took a long walk.

At noon—Packing-sheet, one hour, and bath ten minutes.

Afternoon—The same.

Bandaged throat and chest day and night.

Chronic Sore Throat.—Child two and a half years old. Morning—Packing-sheet one hour and then cold bath; noon, tepid sitz-bath, fifteen minutes.

Bandage round the throat at night, but not by day; rub the throat often with wet hands.

Sore Throat, Pain in the Limbs, and Prostration of Strength.—A young lady so attacked was ordered not to eat any dinner that day; to run up and down stairs and about the room until warm.

Then a blanket, warmed by the fire and the patient enveloped in it, covered by many others, patient to keep in movement in the blanket the first quarter of an hour, to promote perspiration (the sweating process). Bandage throat, chest, and waist. Hold water in the mouth, and rub the throat often with wet hands (requisites in all cases where the throat is engaged). Patient being under the general treatment at the usual time, packing sheet and tepid bath, etc., were used.

Cure effected the second day.

Cold and Cough.—A child six years old. Tepid bath 64° twice a day, fifteen minutes each time, and waist bandage. Cured the second day.

For an adult the above is also good treatment, with the addition of holding water constantly in the mouth when walking, and wearing bandages on chest and legs up to the fork at night; morning, two rubbing sheets; the same at mid-day and in the afternoon. Two foot-baths during the day of ten minutes each; feet to be rubbed well the whole time. Bandages as in former case.

Cold, and Sore Throat.—Bandage the throat at night, expose it by day, even in winter.

Pain in the Bowels.—Packing-sheet until hot, then tepid bath 66° morning and afternoon; at mid-day, sitz-bath 64° twenty minutes. It was truly astonishing to witness the result of one day's treatment.

In a case of great swelling in the throat, bandages were applied to it always, and changed every twenty minutes. To this were added rubbing-sheets three times a day, and a sitz-bath 64° for twenty minutes.

Cold.—In a severe cold, suspend packing-sheet in the morning and substitute rubbing sheet; at noon, packing-sheet for an hour, followed by tepid-bath 64°.

If not soon well, sweating process for an hour and half, followed by tepid bath 64°.

In a common cold, Priessnitz ordered three rubbing-sheets, with great friction, on going to bed. For children, he finds a tepid bath, for ten minutes twice a day, is sufficient; dining on farinaceous food and going out as usual.

Cold with Head Ache.—Two rubbing-sheets and tepid sitz-bath for twenty minutes before dinner, and the same in the afternoon. After each operation a cold-head bath for ten minutes.

Cold, Sore Throat, and enlarged Tonsils.—Packing-sheets and tepid-bath twice a day. Tepid sitz-bath and bandages are generally ordered.

Cold settled in the Knee.—One day rising from kneeling, a patient, aged 50, felt great pain in her knee, which swelled so as to prevent her going out. Despite medical skill, it increased in size, and the foot lost all sensation; this took place twelve months previous to going to Gräfenberg.

The patient for the first seven or eight weeks was confined entirely to her room. In the morning, packing-sheet and tepid bath; noon, stood on the leg up to the top of the thigh in cold water half an hour; afternoon, repeated the same; drank ten glasses of water daily; and kept the leg and foot constantly bandaged. At length she began to walk with two sticks; then she took a cold bath in the morning, and after ten weeks the douche twice a day, ten minutes each time. Digestion good.

The bone resumed its position and the swelling began to diminish; when, the foot having gained its action, she could walk with a stick without other assistance. This lady was an excellent example of the benefit of the Water-cure.

Cough, Sore Throat, and pain in the Chest.—Heating bandage to the throat at night; expose it by day.

Morning, packing-sheet until quite hot; then tepid bath 64° for fifteen minutes twice a day.

In the middle of the day tepid sitz-bath, twenty minutes. It was astonishing to witness the change for the better, after the first day's treatment.

Cold and Cough.—An infant aged six years. Tepid bath 64° twice a day, for fifteen minutes each time.

Heating bandage round the waist. Cured in two days.

Severe Swelling in the Throat.—A gentleman resident in my house was ordered three rubbing-sheets, three times a day, and bandages, changed every twenty minutes.

A friend of mine was constantly annoyed by relaxed and sore throat, without any assignable cause. At length it was found that he slept with his mouth open. An Indian-rubber band to go under the chin and over the head, so as to keep his mouth shut was used at nights and from that time he was no more annoyed with the complaint.

Flatulency.—Injection and sitz-baths.

Drowsiness.—Foot-bath, and rub the head with wet hands. If these means are not sufficient, use the packing-sheet, followed by friction in tepid bath for an hour.

A patient complaining to Priessnitz of feeling heavy in the head after dinner, was ordered to pour a bottle of water on his head, and take head-baths occasionally.

Hysteria.—Rubbing-sheets every five minutes, until every appearance of hysteria is gone. The patient should lie in bed between each packing-sheet to get warm.

Ague.—Tepid bath 62° with great friction until fever is reduced; then packing-sheets, changed on becoming warm; followed by tepid bath, bandage, drinking water, etc. The sweating stage is much relieved by packing-sheets.

Shivering.—For a shivering fit, a patient was ordered five rubbing-sheets, with an interval of five minutes between them—patient to walk about the room during that time: first application effected a cure.

A young lady strong and robust, always cold, sleepy, and indisposed to leave the house, was ordered to use the packing-sheet until warm; then a tepid bath for an hour and upwards, three times a day. In three days she was perfectly well.

Weakness of Chest and Short Breathing.—A delicate lady was ordered two packing-sheets, from the arm-pits to knees, and tepid bath 64°. Feet being cold were rubbed in shallow foot-bath for a quarter of an hour, then dried, and she walked about her chamber for a quarter of an hour before going to bed.

Itching of the Fingers, like the approach of Chilblains.—Wash hands in tepid water, 64°, three times a day for five minutes; wear heating-bandage from the wrist to the elbow.

XLVII.—Sore Mouth—Inflamed Gums.

For this complaint, sweating twice a day, long tepid baths, head-baths, and sitz-baths, were ordered. Tepid water, 68°, should be held in the mouth.

XLVIII.—Tooth-ache, Preservation of the Teeth, etc.

If the tooth is unsound, it must be stopped or extracted. Sometimes when a tooth is plugged, the pressure on the nerve renders it insupportable. At Geneva, a clever dentist avoided this painful result by first cleaning out the tooth, then placing a small plate of metal very flat and thin as a sort of shelf in the tooth, so as to leave a hollow below it. By this means, he avoided the pressure upon the nerve, and the stopping was not felt. This is foreign to our purpose; but I insert it as a useful hint. In ordinary cases of tooth-ache, or inflammation of the gums, fill the mouth with warm water; then with the hand dipped frequently in cold water, rub the cheeks until it can be borne no longer; then rub the gums even to bleeding, and bandage the face: if pain returns in the night, repeat the rubbing. Long and often-repeated tepid foot-baths are also useful.

A patient at Gräfenberg writes as follows:—"Priessnitz ordered me, for tooth-ache and pain in my gums, to rub the back of my head and down my neck often and for a long time. The first application afforded me relief. After ten or fifteen minutes' rubbing, the pain would leave for hours, and then return. Soon there was a longer interval between the attacks: at last, the pain ceased altogether." The theory of this mode of curing such an ailment is based upon true philosophical principles. Who does not know that the nerves of the teeth centre in the back of the head? It is evident, then, that by friction to that part, the inflammation will be drawn from the gums.

A friend of mine, suffering intensely from pain in the gums, found relief from a tepid sitz-bath of thirty minutes. As a preservative for the teeth, there is nothing like water. It is related in a useful little pamphlet, entitled "Facts, proving Water to be the only beverage fitted to give health and Strength to Man," that General Norton, the Mohawk Chief, who was in this country some years ago, said that when the Indians are in their own settlements, living upon the produce of the chase, and drinking water, their teeth always look clean and white; but when they go into the United States, and get spirituous liquors, their teeth look dirty and yellow, and then they are frequently afflicted with tooth-ache, and are obliged to have their teeth drawn. For cleaning the teeth and preserving them, there is nothing so good as cold water; warm or tepid water exposes us to catch cold in the gums, whilst those who are in the constant habit of using cold water are seldom troubled in this way.

XLIX.—Watery or Inflamed Eyes.

For watery eyes, an eye-bath three times a day for five minutes will draw blood to, and strengthen, them. For inflamed eyes, throw water with the hand into them three times a day for five minutes each time, and wear a bandage on the forehead at night.

Sore Eyes.—Place the back part of the head in cold water three times a day, ten minutes each time; then use an eye-bath for five minutes, twice a day: for this purpose, glasses are to be procured of the form of the eye. After the eyes are closed in the water for about a minute, they should be opened for the other four minutes. At night, a bandage should be placed at the back of the neck: this and the head-bath have the effect of drawing inflammation from the front. In most cases, foot-baths twice a day are beneficial. Where there is great inflammation; a very wet bandage may be applied to the eyes for an hour occasionally. As a preservative to the eyes, open them in the wash-hand basin of a morning for two minutes, or throw water [i]nto them occasionally, for two or three minutes at a time.

L.—Deafness.

Rubbing-Sheet three times a day, wear bandage over the ears at night, and drink plentifully of water; tepid sitz-baths. This treatment will often relieve deafness: where it is ineffectual, the general treatment must be resorted to.

LI.—Ear-Ache.

Linen wetted should be introduced into the ear; all round the ear often rubbed with wet hands for a quarter of an hour each time, and a bandage worn round the head; also tepid foot-bath for half an hour.

In obstinate cases, perspiration and tepid baths, sitz and foot-baths, must be resorted to. For an obstinate pain in the ear in a strong man, two packing-sheets and tepid bath for two hours were prescribed; next day, sweating for five or six hours, and cold bath.

LII.—Ringworm, Itch, etc.

These diseases are more easily conquered by Hydropathy than by any other means. The most difficult ringworms to cure, are those driven in by bad treatment. This disease is equal to gout in obstinacy. We shall here warn the sufferer that the diet prescribed must be rigorously observed. Dr. Munde states that "three men, attacked with this disease, arrived at Gräfenberg, at the same time as himself; the first, following the treatment with energy for two months, returned home resolved to continue through the winter, and then return to Gräfenberg to finish the cure, which, at the time of his departure, was more than half effected. The two others remained at Gräfenberg, one for eight months, the other six; both left radically cured. The treatment of one of these cases was attended by an acidity in the throat, and by the vomiting of matter containing chalky substances. The acidity of the throat was such, that it caused the tongue to be ulcerated.["]

LIII.—Psoriasis.

The following extraordinary case is as stated by the patient, an English gentleman, himself. An eruption made its appearance on his head when twenty-three years of age; cause unknown. Underwent medical treatment six years, and tried every remedy five physicians could suggest. Thrice salivated, tried all sorts of ointments, some so powerful as to burn the flesh. Visited Harrowgate the third time, when the eruption spread all over his body. Stomach and bowels a continual source of annoyance. Arrived at Gräfenberg 27th July, 1843; next morning, went into tepid, from that to cold, and back to tepid bath; and afterwards pursued the following treatment:—

Morning, two packing-sheets, the first for a quarter of an hour, the second for an hour, followed by tepid bath for half a minute, then cold, and back to tepid bath; noon, packing-sheet one hour, and rubbing-sheet; afternoon, packing-sheet one hour, and rubbing-sheet. At the expiration of first bath, the bowels acted regularly. Morning and afternoon treatment the same; noon, douche three minutes, and sitz-bath half an hour.

Sept. 5.—Considerable pain felt in thighs and legs; ordered after douching to walk a few minutes, with legs exposed to the air.

Sept. 20.—Diarrhœa. For this, the patient was put into packing-sheet doubled, from the arm-pits to the hips till warm; this was renewed seven times every quarter of an hour. Patient free from pain, but weak. Cramp returned in the evening, when a tepid sitz-bath was ordered, if that did not succeed, a clyster was to be administered.

The sitz-bath removed the pain. About this time pain in his side, which patient had felt from his youth, left him and has not returned. Patient observed that the smell of the packing-sheets, after his having lain in them, was offensive. Eruption at this time evidently worse. Third month, packing-sheet and cold bath instead of tepid bath, and in the afternoon cold bath instead of rubbing-sheet.

Reaction after every operation improved. Eruption so bad that skin cracked in various places, and discharged yellow gummy matter.

Fourth month.—Eruption caused head to feel quite sore; wore bandage to head and changed it four times a day.

Fifth month.—Rheumatic pains in shoulder, which had been felt at intervals for years. Rubbed well on coming out of cold bath; pain ceased in eight or ten days. After some time the pain returned again in both shoulders; this was subdued by rubbing-sheets as follows:—three the same night on going to bed; next day at noon, four afternoon, packing-sheet, followed by three rubbing-sheets, and on going to bed five more. Never felt rheumatic pain since. Eruption worse, covering the entire surface of head and ears, and spots on the body as before.

Jan. 8.—Ceased sweating from weakness; eruption improved in appearance.

Seventh month.—Commenced sweating again; eruption improved.

Eighth month.—Eruption still improving, leaving the skin inflamed and contracted; the spot on left leg gone, and lumps on neck decreasing in size.

Ninth month.—Head and ears better, left off venturing to expose them to the air; washed them frequently with cold water; eruption began to peel off when rubbed. Towards the end of the month, body quite free from all eruption. Patient winds up by saying, "I have gradually left off the various operations, preparatory to my departure, and am happy to say, that now every particle and sign of the eruption has disappeared."

June 17, 1844.—In a letter written some time afterwards to a friend, he stated that he was perfectly cured of the disease.

Fistula.—Patient three years previously had been cured of stricture, to the treatment for which he attributes his present complaint. Morning, packing-sheet till warm, and cold bath; noon, rubbing-sheet and tepid sitz-bath ten minutes; afternoon, packing-sheet and cold bath. Bandages to the fork and arms, and round the waist always.

In three months, douche for three or four minutes. Sitz-bath to be cold instead of tepid, and alternate days foot-bath and tepid half bath, without rubbing-sheet. Cured in five months.

In three months, douche for three or four months; sitz-bath to be cold instead of tepid; and alternate days foot-bath and tepid half bath, without rubbing-sheet. Cured in five months.

Another patient stated that, he suffered from piles; for these he was drugged and leeched at the anus; treatment which was no doubt the cause of the fistula.

Nose Frost-bitten.—Chafe it with tepid-water 62°, and wear bandage continually.

Leprosy.—Patient ordered three packing-sheets and tepid-baths daily, wet linen drawers and waistcoat, with dry ones over them at night. Another patient wore two pairs of wet drawers for the same disease by day.

In another case, patient was ordered packing-sheets and long cold baths, and slept in a wet dress that fitted him, with a dry one over it; the whole being covered with a thick blanket. The patient described that his dress very soon became dry, whilst the blanket was wet and he was cold. To obviate this, Priessnitz told him to put on a second blanket, and in two hours take it off.

LIV.—Fistula.

Where parties are otherwise in tolerable health, this complaint is always curable in about eight or nine months. When health is established, contractility takes place. In cases where patients have been long under medical treatment, the cure of fistula requires great patience and perseverance.

Morning, packing-sheet and bath; noon, rubbing-sheet, douche; afternoon, four o'clock, douche; five o'clock, packing-sheet and bath.

Bandage to waist and part affected. The latter made of old linen.

Cold food is better for this complaint than hot. No sitz-baths.

LV.—Hæmorrhage, Irregular Menstruation, Pains in the Womb, &c.

All these diseases are successfully combated by hydropathy.

Away from Priessnitz, excessive menstruation requires cautious treatment. Persons so afflicted may, however, adopt the following means of relief.

At the period, wear a large bandage round the waist, wash the body with cold water on rising in the morning.

Drink plentifully of cold water.

When discharge has ceased, use a sitz-bath for fifteen minutes, once or twice a day.

If patient is very ill she must remain in bed lightly covered, wearing a very broad bandage, which must be changed every five minutes, or at most, every ten minutes, until better.

In cases of flooding, equally broad bandage, very wet, and changed often; also bandage the calves of the legs, and change it every five or ten minutes.

In case of great weakness, a tepid bath of 64° for eight or ten minutes, with much friction, must be resorted to, fresh water being constantly added, and fresh air admitted into the room.

At the period when menstruation is coming on, if in great pain, let the abdomen, feet, and legs, be well rubbed for a long time by hands dipped often in cold water.

Too frequent Menstruation.—This frequently arises from weakness; in that case, the general treatment to fortify the system is requisite.

Three rubbing-sheets a day, drink plentifully of cold water, eat everything cold.

On rising in the morning, wash internal parts well with a sponge. If this is not sufficient, add packing-sheet and cold bath in the morning, and during the week, take two tepid sitz-baths fifteen minutes, 62°, rubbing the abdomen all the time. Change waist bandage often.

Irregular Menstruation.—A lady, apparently in good health, came to Gräfenberg in 1840. She suffered greatly from head-aches, occasioned by irregular menstruation; when she arrived, though catamenia was strong, she was ordered a sitz-bath, when it ceased and returned in fourteen days. During the patient's stay, it returned three times, notwithstanding which the treatment was continued.

Sweating morning and evening two hours, followed by first tepid and then cold bath.

During the day two tepid sitz-baths, followed immediately by tepid foot-baths, fifteen minutes each.

Douche three minutes. Head-bath, five minutes each side, making fifteen minutes.

Ten to twelve glasses of water, used waist bandages, and took much exercise. *Cured in six weeks.*

Suppressed Menstruation.—When catamenia comes on, except in extraordinary cases, all the operations of the Water-cure are suspended, but when patients are in a crisis or fever, they are continued. When menstruation, from any cause, is suppressed, the following treatment is prescribed.

Three or four times a day, three or four rubbing-sheets, not much wrung out, with great friction. These are each time to be followed by tepid foot-baths of fifteen minutes each.

A lady at Gräfenberg, for this complaint, took packing-sheet and tepid bath in the morning, four rubbing-sheets at noon, four in the afternoon, and four at night; between each rubbing-sheet, she walked or ran naked about the room, with the windows open, though in the depth of a Silesian winter. This treatment brought on catemenia the third day. No bandage was used. If blood had gone to the head, then foot-baths were to have been applied, and the feet and legs rubbed with hands dipped in water the whole time. If these means had failed, then the sitz-bath and douche were to have been added to the treatment. After every operation, patient must go out of doors and take much exercise, and drink not less than twelve glasses of water a day. In some cases, cold foot-baths are more active than tepid ones; and in obstinate complaints of this kind, the sweating process is useful.

Pains in the Womb.—Tepid sitz-bath from forty minutes to an hour, rubbing the abdomen well whilst in the bath with wet hands. Sweating in cold weather beneficial; in hot weather the contrary. To effect a cure, the general health must be established.

Hæmorrhage, Irregular Menstruation, &c.—A patient aged 42, was cured of hæmorrhage in six minutes.

Packing-sheet followed by rubbing-sheet, were first resorted to. After three weeks it became necessary to increase the packing-sheets to fifty a day. They were applied from the arm-pits down to the hips. Patient kept in a perfect state of repose.

In five days this treatment stopped the hæmorrhage; then packing-sheets and cold baths twice a day, were had recourse to, until patient was cured. No sitz-baths. Large bandage, often renewed, was always worn round the waist.

An English lady of title, nearly exhausted from violent hæmorrhage, arrived at Gräfenberg in October. She was ordered not to put her foot to the ground for two months, to sleep with her window open, and to be covered with one sheet only. After the packing-sheets, she was carried to the cold bath and back to bed. She felt as in an ice-house. In two months, great improvement: then, though winter, and the ground was covered with snow, she was ordered to go out without bonnet or umbrella, and as lightly clad as possible; and to douche twice a day for ten minutes. Everything being done to cause contraction. In May she was declared perfectly cured. The husband, on coming to her, was in ecstasies at her healthy appearance, and was at a loss to find words to express his gratitude to Priessnitz.

Head-ache, Pain in the Limbs, and great uneasiness.—A child taken in the night with the above symptoms accompanied with fever, was ordered immediately—

Rubbing-sheet, sitz-bath, and head-bath; at noon, rubbing-sheet and sitz-bath; afternoon, packing-sheet twenty minutes, and tepid-bath.

If the packing-sheet heated soon, then to be changed for twenty minutes.

If symptoms continued, renew the rubbing-sheets, sitz, and head-baths, in the night.

Patient well in the afternoon.

Pain in the Breast.—A lady, two days after her confinement, had her breast hardened by milk, so that she could not endure the infant's attempt to draw it. She applied the bandage, covered with a dry one; it was immediately soothing, and in less than an hour, the milk began to flow.

The Whites.—These find a certain cure in hydropathy. Very often sitz-bath, beginning with tepid water and afterwards using cold and injections, effect the object. When they do not, rubbing sheet and the douche are resorted to.

A case within my knowledge was cured by the following treatment:

Three tepid sitz-baths 60° daily; morning, two packing sheets; one fifteen minutes, the other twenty-five minutes, followed by cold bath, with cold water thrown over the body; afternoon, the sheets were repeated, and either a rubbing sheet or cold bath. When patient did not feel well the tepid bath was used. Body bandage worn always.

LVI.—Change of Life in Females.

Health would be re-established by a few months' treatment—such as rubbing-sheets and douche; drinking water and wearing the bandage. Those who cannot *devote time* to go to Gräfenberg, should take a rubbing sheet every morning, wear a waist bandage, and drink seven or eight tumblers of water a-day.

LVII.—Treatment of Ladies.

Pain at the Chest, Dry Cough, Weak Digestion, Pain and Pressure at the Nape of the Neck, Cold Feet, Great Emaciation and Suppression of Catemenia for three months, Skin dry and hard, Unable to Walk.—A lady, 38 years of age, for the above symptoms, was treated as follows:—

Morning, packing-sheet and tepid-bath; noon, rubbing-sheet; afternoon, as in the morning.

Bandages on chest and abdomen day and night.

Ten glasses of water drank daily.

In ten days able to walk a little, cough eased, better spirits.

In a month, skin softer; and shortly after, a cold plunge-bath was ordered instead of tepid.

Accouchement.—Experience has demonstrated the utility of cold ablutions, sitz-baths, simple diet, and exercise in the air, to females enceinte; water should be substituted for all stimulants. Madame Priessnitz, for her easy and prompt accouchements, is indebted to cold water and sitz-baths, which she took daily for six weeks previous.

The following statement to me in writing, by an American gentleman, shews the value that ought to be set on hydropathy by ladies.

"From 1837 to 1844 inclusive, Mrs. —— was, to all appearance, very healthy, but had an abortive accouchement every year, sometimes twice a year. After the second accident of this nature, she took advice; when, on one occasion, she was subjected to depletion; another, she was advised to pass her time entirely in a recumbent position; she had the best advice that could be procured in Boston, Florence, and Liverpool. These mishaps caused her many distressing and alarming symptoms. She now went to a hydropathic establishment for a few weeks, and derived great benefit from the treatment; this determined her on going to Gräfenberg, when Priessnitz assured her, if confined there, no doubt need be entertained of a favourable result, or the life of the infant. In April, 1845, she arrived at Gräfenberg; after six weeks she became unwell, and continued so for some time; she, however, persevered in the full treatment until April, 1846, when she gave birth to a male child weighing twelve pounds, six ounces.

"Her treatment had been packing-sheet and cold bath in the morning, rubbing-sheets, douche, and sitz-baths in the after part of the day, all the winter. The latter she took the very morning of her accouchement.

"During labour, the bandages round the waist were quite wet, and changed every ten minutes. She was also ordered to walk and use her arms as much as possible.

"After the birth, she was washed twice a day with tepid water 15°, with wet towels.

"The child, immediately on entering the world, was put into water as it came from the fountain; afterwards warm water was mixed with it until it reached 15°. The child's baths were afterwards tepid 15°, and gradually reduced to 12°. After two months he had two of these baths a day.

"In case of pain in the bowels bandages were applied; if not attended with immediate relief, a cold clyster. He is now three years old, strong and cheerful; his mother free from all those symptoms hitherto so obstinate, mysterious, and apparently fatal. I leave Gräfenberg with the highest sense of gratitude towards the wonderful man, whose intuitive genius has proved such a blessing to thousands. I regard hydropathy a thousand times more as a science of life than a remedial agent. I have seen enough to convince me that he who lives according to its precepts, *must*, barring accidents and pestilence, live to a good old age; it will teach all to make their passions harmonise with their organisation, and then it will be, not only a medicine, but a religion."

If fever of any kind supervenes upon accouchements, wet sheets and tepid-baths are resorted to.

Pregnancy.—A delicate lady, who accompanied her husband to Gräfenberg, became in the family-way; she had long suffered from derangement of the stomach, which now became much worse: she wasted away and became weakly.

Ordered two rubbing-sheets daily, one in the morning, the other in the afternoon. A sitz-bath occasionally.

Bandage round the waist, always drank plentifully of water.

Under this treatment, she became stout and plump. She walked until the day before her accouchement. When she felt the pains of labour coming on, Priessnitz caused her to sit up until the last moment, with a bandage round the abdomen, which, during labour, was changed every six minutes. The delivery was quick and easy.

Experience shews the utility of cold ablutions and exercise in the open air, to females who are in the family-way. To this add simple diet, and drinking plentifully of cold water. All stimulants should be avoided. A sitz-bath occasionally, and a bandage when sensations of pain are felt, will also be beneficial.

Sterility.—I could enumerate instances out of number, of parties (who had often deplored the absence of children) having families, after undergoing the cleansing and fortifying process of the Water-cure.

A gentleman, now an M.P., and his lady, were travelling for their health in Italy. A friend of mine at Venice, advised them to go to Gräfenberg. They did so, and after five months, the lady became enceinte. She wrote afterwards, that she had been married eleven years without having had a child; that since her trip to Gräfenberg she had three. Her meeting with that gentleman at Venice, she said she looked upon as an act of divine Providence.

Difficulty in passing Urine.—Wash the parts with cold water often; the body twice a-day; bandage the parts; drink plentifully of water and eat grapes.

LVIII.—Giddiness, Dizziness, etc.

Bandage (wet) round the head; lie in bed and change body-bandage often. Tepid sitz-bath 62° for forty minutes. If after a few hours, patient is not better, resort to packing-sheet and tepid bath; or three or four rubbing-sheets twice or thrice a-day, followed by tepid foot-baths.

LIX.—Head-Aches.

When they proceed from nervousness, rubbing-sheet for three or four minutes, well wetting the head first, followed by sitz-bath for fifteen minutes. When these fail, resort to packing-sheet and tepid bath. Head-bandage.

It frequently happens that well washing the head, rubbing the temples for a long time with wet hands, and wearing a wet bandage as a turban, the head-ache is relieved.

Head-ache and Flushing from anxiety.—A lad was ordered:

Foot-bath twenty minutes; feet very much rubbed during that time. Body bandaged and bandage often changed.

Tepid sitz-bath 62° quarter of an hour; head-bath for ten minutes, and afterwards bandage round it very often terminates head-ache at once.

When head-ache is obstinate, the duration of the sitz-bath must be extended, and a perpetual bandage from the ankle to the knee. This, though it may produce an eruption, may be continued for months. Bandage the head night and day.

Head-ache.—For a violent head-ache, Priessnitz ordered the body bandage to be changed every ten minutes. This did not answer—when patient was relieved by the following treatment; a rubbing-sheet for five minutes, and sitz-bath for an hour, the head being bandaged all the time.

A lady of a fine strong constitution, suffering from intense nervous head-ache, was treated as follows:—

Morning, packing-sheet and bath, followed by head-bath, three minutes to each side, and the same to the back, making nine minutes; noon, rubbing-sheet, sitz-bath; afternoon as in the morning. Patient always went without stockings and bonnet. In three months health much improved and headache less frequent.

Head-ache.—Some head-aches are relieved by fomenting the forehead and temples with towels wetted with hot water for half an hour, occasionally washing and rubbing those parts with cold water; when, if not cured, the treatment should be repeated, and afterwards a bandage may be applied.

LX.—Acute Inflammation in the Head, Chest and Abdomen.

Frequent rubbing-sheets; packing-sheets, and sitz-bath, cut short the premonitory stage of the disease. In the event of increase of pain and fever, tepid bath 62 to 64 deg. should be used, and patient kept in it until the axillæ are cold. Packing-sheet, after the lapse of twenty-four, thirty-six, or forty-eight hours, when all inflammatory symptoms have ceased, may be had recourse to. Should these symptoms return, the tepid bath must be repeated, and its duration regulated by circumstances.

LXI.—Chilblains.

Put the part affected in tepid water three times a day for twenty minutes; if the fingers are attacked, apply a bandage from the wrist to the elbow; if the toes, from the ankle to the knee, and wear it night and day.

LXII.—Cold Feet.

When cold, to be well rubbed with wet hands, but *never* put into a bath. To cure cold feet, rubbing-sheet to the whole body, and friction to the feet two or three times a day; after which, walk about room, or passage, or cold wet stones, for ten or fifteen minutes, or until heat has returned. Persons suffering from cold feet, on going to bed at night may use the bandage as follows: first bring heat to the feet by exercise or friction; then put a bandage into cold water, wring it out well, envelope the feet in it, and over that place a thick dry bandage.

LXIII.—Cold Hands And Whitlow.

Rub the hands with snow or cold water and let them dry of themselves; when they are wounded, keep the snow or water away from them. To draw heat or bad matter from the hands, bandage from the wrist to elbow and use elbow-bath, fifteen minutes each time. In ordinary cases of whitlow, rub the finger, hand and wrist often with wet hand, and bandage the finger at night. If obstinate, resort to the same treatment as for cold hands.

LXIV.—Bunnion and Enlarged Glands of Foot and Instep.

A lady aged 45 was ordered—morning, packing-sheet twenty minutes and tepid bath 62°; noon, sitz-bath fifteen minutes; afternoon, rubbing-sheet. Bandage to feet and legs up to the knees at night, and from ankles to knees only by day If the feet are wounded by tight boots, take foot-baths twice a-day and wear a bandage on the feet at night.

LXV.—Depression of Spirits, Head-Ache, etc.

A patient derived immediate relief from the following treatment: morning, packing-sheet half an hour, then tepid bath two minutes, cold three or four minutes, and back to the tepid; noon, rubbing-sheet, sitz-bath fifteen minutes and head-bath ten minutes; afternoon, morning treatment repeated. When better, the packing-sheet in the afternoon was abandoned for a sitz-bath ten minutes. On dreary wet days the packing-sheet was to be resorted to again. After the sitz-bath, the feet were to be put into water for two or three minutes and well rubbed.

LXVI.—Deafness.

Away from Gräfenberg, persons are recommended to use the rubbing-sheet twice a-day, take a foot-bath ten minutes, and wear a bandage round the ears at night.

A young man from Hambro', suffering from deafness, followed up the general treatment for three or four months, when a boil appeared on his abdomen and increased to the size of an egg; this burst whilst patient was taking the douche: from that time he heard as well as ever.

LXVII.—Hernia and Constipation.

Both these complaints, which are so completely out of the reach of drugs, are always cured by hydropathy.

Don——, late minister from a foreign court to England, through my interpretation, inquired of Priessnitz how long he should be before he was cured of constipation? A twelvemonth. How long of my hernia? Four months. His treatment was as follows:—

Morning, packing-sheet and tepid bath, afterwards changed to cold bath; noon, rubbing-sheet and sitz-bath; afternoon, as in the morning; bandage to the hernia and round the waist always.

In about four months hernia was perfectly cured and patient declared that as he eat, slept, and walked well, he considered himself in health, and consequently left Gräfenberg. I heard from him in Rome afterwards, when he continued perfectly satisfied.

Hernia.—A German baron, thirty-five years of age, assured me that nine months before I made his acquaintance, he came to Gräfenberg for hernia: that he had been cured the last two months, but he was waiting to be assured of it.

He was induced to come, from a captain in his regiment having been cured of a double rupture two years before.

Cases *ad infinitum* might be quoted to show the certainty of the Water-cure effecting cures of this nature.

LXVIII.—Liver Complaint, Congestion of Blood in the Head, Enlarged Vein in the Leg.

An English M.D., 70 years of age, was attacked with yellow fever in the tropics, which affected his liver, when indigestion and dyspepsia resulted.

At Rome, being seized with pain in the heart and congestion of blood in the head, he was bled: finding himself no better, he proceeded for the best advice to Paris, where depletion was again recommended. This determined him to go to Gräfenberg.

The doctor told me Priessnitz took a most accurate view of his case: he began by packing-sheets and tepid-bath, morning and evening; rubbing-sheets, sitz and foot-baths at noon.

The treatment caused him varied sensations, but generally a tendency to healthy action. One day he felt unusual pain about the region of the heart, and congestion in the head. Having a gouty tendency in his system, he became alarmed, and sent for Priessnitz, who put a large wet bandage doubled in the form of a shawl over his shoulders, and over the region of the heart, and then requested him to put his feet up to the knees in cold water for half an hour.

The doctor declared to me, that if asked a question as to the danger of such a proceeding, he should have said that he thought death would immediately ensue, and that but for the confidence Priessnitz' success, as witnessed by himself, had created, no power on earth could have induced him in such a complaint to follow the orders thus given. As it was, however, he plunged his feet into the water at once in presence of Priessnitz, who stood with him the whole time. By degrees the symptoms decreased; in an hour after the operation he was completely relieved, and that night slept remarkably well.

For a slight attack of fever, the doctor was prescribed five or six rubbing-sheets and a head-bath, to walk in the open air, and change his body-bandage in the night. At another time, for blood to the head and great nervousness, he bathed the head after dinner, bandaged the neck and dispensed with neck handkerchief.

When the doctor first came to Gräfenberg, his walks were limited to the piazza in front of his rooms; these were extended by degrees, until even during the inclemency of the winter and the depth of snow everywhere encountered, he extended his walks thrice a day up into the woods, and was always the first to be seen out in the morning. In about nine months, the gentleman was completely cured of all his ailments.

LXIX.—Deformity.

An artisan kept his bed for a long time, his illness is supposed to have originated in a cold. He was almost bent double. In this state he went to Carlsbad, where the waters rendered him so weak that he moved about with great difficulty. In this state he came to Gräfenberg.

Morning, packing-sheet one hour, bath three minutes; noon, two rubbing-sheets and sitz-bath; afternoon as the morning.

Large bandage round the loins, drank twenty tumblers of water before breakfast; and twenty more during the day.

In about three months this patient was able to ascend the highest hills, then he was ordered to carry loads of wood on his head, and put a stick behind his back through his arms at all times, to assist in bringing him straight. He staid all the winter: in the spring his health was perfect, and he was nearly upright when I left him at Gräfenberg.

LXX.—Spinal Complaints.

Priessnitz says it is difficult to prescribe for these complaints at a distance; and that except in young people, or where the disease is in its infancy, a cure is seldom effected. It is however always safe to adopt the following treatment, which will refresh and strengthen the patient.

Three rubbing-sheets, at intervals during the day.

One or two foot-baths, but NO sitz-baths without advice.

If the feet swell, continue the treatment, all the same, rub with wet hands, and bandage the legs, from the ankle to the knee, this will reduce the swelling.

Spine complaint and general debility.—A lady.

Morning, packing-sheet until warm, followed by plunge-bath one minute; noon, douche three minutes, return home and then take a rubbing-sheet and sitz-bath, twenty minutes; afternoon, as in the morning.

Rubbed the back and nape of the neck with wet hands, twice a day.

Patient staid all the winter; during which time symptoms were combated as they arose, she gained strength and flesh.

Spinal affection.—A young lady, after submitting to all sorts of medical treatment for three or four years, came to Gräfenberg. She was clothed in flannel, suffered greatly from indigestion, constipation, and languid circulation, feet always cold, walking a short distance brought on pain in the back.

Second day after her arrival, Priessnitz ordered,—

"Put aside all flannel, go as lightly clad as possible, keep bed-room window open day and night, and sleep with only a single sheet as a covering, leave off stockings and run bare-footed on the wet grass near the house, or on the cold stones of the passage for half an hour before breakfast in the morning.

"Eat black bread and drink sour milk, lie on the stomach and have the spine rubbed several times a day with wet hands."

First four days, patient had cold feet in and after the packing-sheet, this was then followed by tepid, then cold, and back to tepid-bath, feet well rubbed, previous to going into packing-sheet, and last thing at night; by this treatment head-ache was relieved and the feet became warmer.

In ten days began the douche for one minute; digestion improved; no longer constipated. Bandages always round the body, and to feet and legs at night.

Patient was at Gräfenberg nine months, during which time the treatment was often changed to meet circumstances. One time, suppressed catamenia was relieved in two days by sixteen rubbing-sheets a day. At another, patient met with an accident in the leg; Priessnitz to keep this to the surface, ordered more water to be drunk. This patient left Gräfenberg in excellent health, though not entirely cured of the affection of the spine, that being out of its perpendicular position.

Pain in the Shoulder and Chest.—A lady in the treatment complained of pain in the shoulder and left breast, and down the side.

Ordered, when in sitz-bath the upper part of the body to be well rubbed.

Body bandage to be more wrung out than usual, and extra covering over it.

Pain in the side, Chronic cold in the head.—A German officer aged 50, afflicted as above, and with continued stoppage in the nose, and frequent head-aches, was told by his medical man that he had no chance of being cured, was completely relieved at Gräfenberg, in three or four months.

Packing-sheets and tepid baths twice a day. Rubbing-sheet and sitz-baths were resorted to for a short time, the cold bath substituted for the tepid bath, and to this treatment the douche was added.

Weak Chest and Worms.—A child three years old. Wash with tepid water, 12° once, and after some time twice a day.

Wear body bandage always, and drink water.

Pain in the Chest.—A gentleman had pain in his chest, like the hurt from a blow, about the size of a crown-piece.

Ordered sixteen rubbing-sheets a day, *four at each time.*

LXXI.—Constipation.

This complaint is always relieved, and if sufficient time is devoted to the treatment, finally overcome by Hydropathy; space forbids my going into details, or numerous cases might be given in proof of this assertion. The reader's attention may however be called to the letter addressed to a newspaper, and signed by upwards of one hundred patients, giving the case of the son of Prince Leichtenstein, who was cured in a few days of Constipation, which had endured twenty-eight days in defiance of all medical aid. To effect a permanent cure, the treatment must be persevered in for a long time, very often a twelvemonth.

In a recent case. Rubbing-sheets until feverish heat ceases: sometimes four or three suffice; at others the number must be increased to sixteen or twenty, to be immediately followed by a clyster. Then take a walk, and on returning, a sitz-bath fifteen to twenty minutes, the abdomen to be well rubbed the whole time.

Body bandage to be worn always and often changed. This treatment to be resorted to twice a day. Great exercise to be used, and cold light food to be partaken of.

A delicate lady who had suffered from this complaint for upwards of twenty years, was relieved in a fortnight, and had no return of it during her stay at Gräfenberg. Her principal treatment was:—

Packing-sheet and bath twice a day. Rubbing-sheet and sitz-bath at noon.

A second case, which came under my observation, was that of a Russian, who for many years had only been relieved by medicine or enemas. He went to an establishment at Moscow for six months, where he derived great benefit, though he still used enemas. At Gräfenberg he abandoned the latter, his bowels were relaxed and have continued so ever since.

LXXII.—Indigestion.

Foul tongue and pain at the pit of the stomach; a lady having tried all other remedies, was ordered the following, which answered admirably.

Three cold sitz-baths a day, for an hour each time, rubbing the abdomen the whole time, eat nothing but brown bread and drink sour milk during three days.

Loss of Appetite, Foul Tongue, etc.—Patient had foul tongue, and loss of appetite.

Morning.—Sweating and tepid bath, stomach to be well rubbed in the bath. Sitz-bath thirty minutes in the afternoon.

It is very essential to drink abundantly of water, and take great exercise.

A child five years old. Pale, foul tongue, loss of appetite, thirsty and awaking with screams. Ablution in the morning, and three tepid sitz-baths daily four minutes each; chest, back, and abdomen to [be] well rubbed all the time; waist bandage day night. Drink as much water as possible. Cured in three months.

LXXIII.—Stomach Complaint.

Patient's stomach deranged, food used to return to his mouth: difficult of cure. His second visit to Gräfenberg, cured in nine months. Packing-sheets and rubbing-sheets. Noon, douche, rubbing-sheet and sitz-bath; afternoon, packing-sheet and bath.

LXXIV.—Throwing Food off the Stomach.

Morning, rubbing-sheet and sitz-bath fifteen minutes. Noon, the same repeated. Afternoon, sitz-bath.

A gentleman of my acquaintance pursued three or four months' treatment for this complaint, and left Gräfenberg without being cured.

LXXV.—Heartburn.

Drink large quantit[i]es of water fasting, rub the part with wet hands and wear a large bandage, changed often, round the waist. If this does not effect a cure, take a rubbing-sheet or two and a tepid sitz-bath twice a day. Nausea and sickness are to be treated in the same manner; if, however, the latter become chronic, then packing-sheets, tepid baths, and sitz-baths must be resorted to. The diet should be brown bread and milk only. The milk should be boiled, if it otherwise disagrees with the patient.

LXXVI.—Sea Sickness.

To avoid sea-sickness or relieve it. The traveller should lay on his back, and place a large wet towel on his abdomen, changing it when dry. After a sea voyage take a few rubbing-sheets and sitz-baths. Wear a waist bandage, and if constipated resort to cold water clysters.

LXXVII.—Palpitation of the Heart.

Many rubbing-sheets; rub the whole, side for a long time and often. Large bandage. Two sitz-baths a day, fifteen minutes each; rubbing the afflicted side the whole time. A lady afflicted as above was relieved in ten minutes by the rubbing-sheets, and dabbling her feet well in cold water.

LXXVIII.—Want of Sleep.

Before going to bed, take a shallow foot-bath (only to cover the soles of the foot) for seven to ten minutes, rubbing the feet to above the ankles all the time, then walk about the room bare-footed until the feet are quite warm.

A lady, in the treatment, complained of want of sleep.

Two packing-sheets in the afternoon, the first changed as soon as hot, followed by tepid bath.

Two foot-baths for one hour each, the water only to cover the soles of the feet. Feet to be well rubbed the whole time. When the servant is tired of rubbing, patient should walk about the room with bare feet for a few minutes and then resume the foot-bath.

LXXIX.—Languid Circulation.

I attended many cases of this kind with Mr. Priessnitz, where the languid circulation arose from using the head more than the body. In a general way he began with rubbing-sheets in the morning and afternoon for a few days, and then in the morning packing-sheet until warm, and tepid bath, cold bath, and back to tepid bath. Noon, rubbing-sheet and tepid sitz-bath fifteen minutes; afternoon, packing-sheet and tepid baths as in the morning; or a rubbing-sheet. Bandaged always.

LXXX.—Ring Worm.

A boy aged seven years had ring worm over the eye and behind his knees. Cured in six weeks. Two packing-sheets and tepid baths daily. Bandage to the knees. Child could not endure the douche.

LXXXI.—Hands Frost-bitten or Suffering from a Boil.

Rub the hands well with tepid water, and particularly the wrist. Put the elbow into cold water for twenty minutes, three times a day. Bandage the whole arm from the arm-pits down to the wrist.

LXXXII.—Weak Eyes and Eruption on the Head.

A child two years old had weak eyes, from which there was a constant discharge and an eruption on the face and head; it was treated as follow:—

Packing-sheet one hour and sometimes longer, followed by tepid bath. Large bandage from hips to arm-pits night and day. Dabbed the face often with cold water and bandaged the head at night. In three weeks eyes quite well and the eruption diminished.

LXXXIII.—Weak Ankles.

If an infant, ablution every morning and bandage the ankles night and day. If an older person, ablution and foot-baths twenty minutes. Morning and afternoon, bandage always.

LXXXIV.—Treatment of Infants.

Immediately after birth bathe the infant in warm water 82°, put a wet bandage on navel, bound on with a dry one, change it morning and evening *only*. Continue this until the navel is healed. The temperature of the bath to be reduced two degrees every fortnight, until 68°, which is to be used until child can run alone. It may be washed with cold water at three months of age.

If an Infant is uneasy or restless and cries.—Put on a body bandage; if this is not sufficient, give it an extra tepid-bath.

The child of an Hungarian commissioner was born weak and sickly, with great difficulty in breathing. The physicians treated the mother to improve the milk, when the child refused the breast. From three days old it was spoon-fed. On the fifth or sixth day, the father put the child into a packing-sheet until it was warm, when he changed it, and then applied the tepid-bath.

After four day's treatment a lump appeared on the chest, which increased until it became as large as a man's fist. On the eighth day it broke, and half a tumbler of matter was discharged. From this moment the child gradually improved and is now the healthiest of his children.

Child-teething, Pain in the Head, and Diarrhœa.—Tepid bath for about five minutes three times a day.

Two head-baths from ten to fifteen minutes each, and one clyster.

A body bandage, and change it often.

LXXXV.—Epilepsy.

This complaint in a general way is not to be cured by Hydropathy; but Priessnitz thinks persons subject to it should use cold baths, and cold water as a beverage. I know a young man who was six months at Gräfenberg, it is now twelve-months since, and as he has not had an attack, he considers himself cured.

LXXXVI.—Hypochondria and Hysteria.

A disarrangement of the system, and inaction of the abdomen, cause much uneasiness and discontent. This disease being moral as well as physical, requires pure air, scenery, society, and a complete change in the manner of living. What is so calculated to combat this complaint as Hydropathy?

A patient became hypochondriac, in consequence of chronic derangement of bowels, struck with rush of blood to the head, face became crimson, lost speech and consciousness, had convulsions and spasmodic movement of the arms.

First operation was to put him into a cold bath, and use strong friction for an hour. He was put into a packing-sheet, in which he became delirious; he was then rubbed by four men in a tepid bath, 64°. He was still unconscious and yet winced on being pinched; water thrown on his head caused a slight cry; great heat on the head. On ceasing the cold affusion, pulse though oppressed began to be felt—eyes fixed—conjunctiva inflamed.

Friction continued two hours, then ceased for one hour and a half, and begun again: in an hour spasms ceased, eyes began to move, without seeing.

Patient apparently exhausted, pulse gained its power, though still often intermittent, upper part of the body hot, lower extremities could not be warmed all night, consciousness had not returned in the morning, pulse better, but sleep interrupted,—patient groaning. All night wet bandage applied to the head. At 6 o'clock next morning, sweating process, perspiration preceded consciousness, up to which moment patient was insensible to all that had occurred. After half an hour's sweating, he was well rubbed in tepid bath 66°, and put to bed, when he slept. On awaking he partook of bread and milk.

At 2 o'clock P.M., awoke covered with perspiration, and from that time until next morning, slept at intervals, pulse regular, talked calmly and rationally, bowels in a normal state.

In the morning, packing-sheet; and later, sweating process; both followed by tepid bath 64°—temperature of the body still high. After good night's rest, appetite returned, and so much better as to renew the treatment to effect a cure of that which brought him to Gräfenberg.

LXXXVII.—Fœtid Perspiration of the Feet.

This is relieved by foot-baths, and wearing a bandage on the feet at night; but it cannot be cured without the sweating process.

LXXXVIII.—Stricture.

Sweating and tepid bath, and cold sitz-baths, are generally resorted to in this complaint. If cold water is found too severe, tepid is used for a time; a bandage is always applied to parts affected.

For stoppage of the water, three to six rubbing-sheets; if they fail, resort to sweating process until water comes, then a tepid bath, or rubbing-sheet.

Medical men, to effect this object, put the patient first into a warm bath, and then bleed him until he faints: by these means, the prostate gland becomes relaxed, and water flows; or water is passed by the use of catheters, which at Gräfenberg are always dispensed with.

LXXXIX.—Inflammation of the Kidneys And Urethra.

The treatment must be regulated by circumstances: sometimes sweating, at other times the packing-sheet, tepid bath, and bandage.

XC.—Hydrocephalus.

A child one year and a-half old had water on the brain, and a large protuberance in the middle of the forehead. Ordered, a tepid bath morning and evening; a rubbing-sheet after an hour's sleep at noon, and repeated before going to bed at night. Drank water only at meals, and then but little. Bandage from arm-pits down to the knees; was much in the open air. After twelve months, the protuberance went down, leaving a ridge like a pigeon's breast down the centre; shape of head completely changed, and the boy was perfectly well.

XCI.—Syphilis.

This complaint always succumbs to the treatment; and a cure effected by it leaves none of those lamentable consequences which attend the exhibition of drugs. By Hydropathic means, the virus is completely thrown out of the system through the pores; whilst the administration of mercury is attended with secondary symptoms, which are more fatal than the disease itself. If taken in time, secondary symptoms are also cured at Gräfenberg. It frequently happens, that patients treated for another complaint, find syphilis return, though they imagined themselves cured of it years before. Recent cases of syphilis in otherwise healthy persons, are generally cured in less than two months; but the cure of secondary symptoms is a work of time. There are many sufferers from this undermining malady, who have been at Gräfenberg one, two, and even three years. In health, they, are much improved; but the malady is too deeply seated to be eradicated. One gentleman, when I was there, was refused admittance; he died in a few days, when it was found that mercury had eaten part of his wind-pipe away—a result that never could have been brought about by water. The following is another deplorable case, the result of bad treatment:—Patient aged thirty-five, tall, thin, and bent when walking; supports his head by pressing his hands on each side of it; part of the cranium destroyed. The brain covered over by a skin; the parietal bones destroyed, and thick pus exudes between the skin and bone, and smells horribly. Inside of the left eye is an ulceration with raised borders, which allows a portion of the orbital arch to be seen surrounded with pus; pulse weak and irregular; constant pain. Treated for secondary symptoms, with mercury in 1841; came to Gräfenberg with three ulcers the size of a shilling on his forehead, with burning pains. Packing-sheets and tepid baths morning and evening, with other intermediate treatment. This case is introduced to show the sort of cases Mr. Priessnitz will undertake: of course, a cure will require a considerable time.

XCII.—Chancre.

Case of a very strong young man:—

For five days—sweating (after perspiration broke out) morning, one hour; afternoon, half an hour; then tepid bath, followed by cold bath and back to tepid. After five days—from sweating went into plunging cold bath; in another week, douched from two to five minutes at eleven o'clock; bandage round the body and on the sores, which were bathed and had water thrown on them frequently; wore suspending bandages; eat sparingly; no meat or butter, and took but little exercise. Perfectly cured in six weeks.

XCIII.—Gonorrhœa and Chancres.

Sweating, followed by bath in the morning; douche at eleven; at twelve, rubbing-sheet and sitz-bath; afternoon, packing-sheet and bath; chancres increased to the size of a sixpence then, and in two days cicatrised. Patient cured in twenty-five days.

Gonorrhœa, &c.—Packing-sheet, tepid bath, and sitz-baths were the means used. The complaint continuing, Priessnitz supposed it arose from debility of the parts, and ordered:—

Six sitz-baths of ten minutes, allowing five minutes to elapse between each, twice a-day; packing-sheets to be changed as soon as warm, followed by cold bath.

A young man, immediately on discovering this complaint, who took sitz-baths as above described, injected cold water into the urethra, bandaged the parts and drank plentifully of cold water and lived low; was cured in two days.

Another person was subject to involuntary emissions, by which his strength was wasting away. In a month after he began the cure, he found an old gonorrhœa return (which had evidently been driven into the system and was the cause of his malady); he was now treated for this and restored to perfect health.

A Russian officer, declared cured of chancre three years before, found the complaint return, when he was again treated by mercury. His throat continued to trouble him, his voice was husky, and piles began to make their appearance. After pursuing the Water-cure for a short time, as described in a former case, he had a crisis in his foot, and diarrhœa for a fortnight, when he passed a considerable quantity of blood. After this, the piles disappeared entirely, and his voice became sound and clear. It should be observed that he sweated alternate mornings only; the other mornings, packing-sheets and bath.

A young man aged 23, attacked with secondary symptoms: sore throat, etc., was ordered three packing-sheets and cold baths a-day; rubbing-sheet and sitz-bath.

I knew another strong young man suffering under secondary symptoms, so that he could hardly walk with the use of a stick; he went to Gräfenberg, staid there two months, and returned to England the picture of health.

As there are always at Gräfenberg a large number of individuals labouring under these complaints, cases of cure might be adduced *ad infinitum*: suffice it to say, that hydropathy in their cure is omnipotent. Buboes and chancres, when taken in their infancy, are eradicated from the system in a few weeks, sometimes days, without the debilitating effects attendant upon other deceitful remedies.

XCIV.—Scrofula and Vaccination.

Priessnitz, when asked what he conceived to be the cause of such an increase of scrofula as is said to have taken place of late years, said, he attributed it to vaccination, syphilis and drugs.

When vaccination is performed without producing its desired effect, the virus remains in the system, and when it proceeds favourably, it is a question if it is ever thoroughly ejected.

Every practitioner knows the difficulty that exists of finding children from which to take matter where no taint is in the blood. The child subjected to vaccination is not only exposed to the sins of his own forefathers, but also to those of the stranger.

The consequences attendant upon syphilis, and the evil results of mineral poisons, are such as to lead us to believe that Priessnitz' opinion is not without foundation. I am doubtful whether scrofula is ever cured,[7] though whilst at Gräfenberg I saw many obstinate cases relieved. Children who arrived there perfect cripples, were enabled to use their limbs like other people. I think I may in great truth say, that in all cases the enemy received a check, and the general health of the patient was improved.

A patient states, that previous to inoculation his family were well; but since that operation they have been scrofulous. He came to Gräfenberg some years ago from Dartres, when Priessnitz told him to go home, give up all beverages but water, use cold baths daily, and he would be well; though incredulous, he followed the advice, and in two years was perfectly cured.

For scrofula, the whole treatment must be persevered in for a long time.

XCV.—Piles.

Piles are caused by an accumulation of blood in the vessels which merge into the large intestines; they either discharge blood, or are confined to a swelling of the veins, in otherwise healthy subjects. Hydropathy effects a radical cure of this complaint, whilst medical remedies are only temporary, and often lead to serious consequences.

Treatment.—Morning, three rubbing-sheets and sitz-bath, twenty minutes; noon, the same; afternoon, the same, and an additional sitz-bath, making four sitz-baths during the day. At night, a rubbing-sheet but no sitz-bath, as it is too late to walk after it. Body bandage; much water to be drunk; douche four to eight minutes in the middle of the day, if possible.

Out of the general treatment, persons troubled with piles may take sitz-baths and wear a bandage on the part affected.

A patient having piles and sore eyes, was advised neither to take sitz-baths or eye-baths. When Priessnitz was asked the reason, he said, "Because you have too much bad matter in your system, which I am afraid of attracting to those parts."

In a common attack of piles, two or three sitz-baths a-day, fifteen minutes each, and wearing a bandage upon the part at night, will afford relief.

Persons subject to piles should especially avoid all heating and stimulating drinks.

XCVI.—Rupture.

I knew of a case of double rupture, in an officer 34 years of age, which was perfectly cured at Gräfenberg in three years. Another case of single rupture was cured in nine months, and a recent one cured in four months.

There can be no doubt of the complete omnipotence of Hydropathy over this malady; its cure is only a matter of time. It is difficult to lay down any prescribed treatment, as the chief aim of the practitioner must be to bring his patient into fine health. All organic action is contraction; all strength depends upon the power of the different parts of the body to contract, and nothing will aid the operation so much as the different appliances here made use of. As a rule, I observed that when rupture exudes, the sweating process should be resorted to; when perspiration has broken out, gently rub the part with the hand until the rupture is gone in again. Bandages are worn continually.

XCVII.—Chilblains.

Rub the feet or hands affected for a quarter of an hour in tepid water three times a-day, and bandage the leg from ankle to knee if in the feet. If in the hand, the arm from wrist to elbow.

XCVIII.—Cold Feet.

Take a shallow foot-bath, cold, one inch deep, before going to bed, for fifteen minutes; let the feet be well rubbed the whole time, then walk about the room bare-footed for half an hour, so that re-action may take place, or they will be colder than before.

XCIX.—Eruption, Scabs, and Sores on the Arms.

A child had tried sulphur bandages and all other conceivable means:—

Morning, noon, and afternoon, packing-sheet and tepid-bath; the latter after a few days changed to the cold-bath; bandages night and day; cure effected in a few weeks.

C.—Consumption.

Until the age of fifteen or sixteen Priessnitz conceives this complaint to be always curable. Very often when parties are supposed to be consumptive, they are not so. A young lady arrived at Gräfenberg during my stay there. I thought she had delayed it too long; she appeared in the last stage of consumption. Priessnitz however took the case—and, principally with rubbing-sheets, administered three times a-day, effected an extraordinary cure in two months. I saw this lady afterwards at Florence, and was quite surprised to see what an extremely fine woman she had become.

There was also a young lady suffering under the following symptoms:— great debility, very thin, weak eyes, little or no appetite, and a short cough, which would awaken her about four o'clock in the morning, and trouble her the whole day. She was considered by M.D.'s as consumptive. Priessnitz took a different view of the case, and as she was cured in two months he was right. Her treatment was as follows:—

Morning, packing-sheet and plunge bath, the tepid-bath having been used only for a short time; at ten o'clock, douche; at eleven, rubbing-sheet and eye-bath; at five, packing-sheet and bath; chest, waist, and forehead bandaged every night; waist bandaged always.

Consumption of the Nerves.—A gentleman aged 30, came to Gräfenberg in a most deplorable state, supported on one side by his wife, on the other by his servant. Second night he was taken alarmingly ill, with a fever and a stoppage in his bowels. He was too weak for a packing-sheet or tepid-bath, therefore twelve rubbing-sheets were administered within three hours; and two head-baths during the intermediate times. When a change for the better took place, enemas were applied and relief afforded. The next day patient was out of doors. I left Gräfenberg about this time, therefore do not know if he recovered.

Spitting Blood.—A young lady was subjected to spitting blood, pain at the chest, and general debility. Priessnitz doubted if the lungs were affected, and tried packing-sheet and tepid-bath, which patient was found too weak to support. Then rubbing-sheets twice a day; patient still too weak. Then rubbing-sheet, and tepid sitz-bath ten minutes. Feverish excitement and loss of appetite came on. Back of head put into cold water for quarter of an hour; to be repeated several times a day. Bandage at all times down the middle of the breast and round the waist. When spitting of blood came on, then cold foot-baths were resorted to. Patient tried the treatment for a month, but was not much improved by it.

On leaving, Priessnitz advised her to spend the winter in Italy, to eat nothing but bread and grapes, and to use cold ablutions.

CI.—Insanity.

This disease, Priessnitz says is curable, when it proceeds from bodily suffering or disease; but when caused by mental suffering or misfortune, is generally incurable. I witnessed the treatment of a case of aberration of mind at Gräfenberg; the patient was put into a tepid-bath, held there, and rubbed for nine hours and a half; he was then put to bed, and next morning awoke perfectly composed.

Hydrophobia.—Dr. Short in 1656, published a work, in which he stated, that with cold water, he had cured the bite of mad dogs and dropsy. Priessnitz says he never treated the human subject for this complaint, but that he had cured a dog, by tying him up and throwing a large number of pails of water over him. At first it caused him to shiver a great deal, proving the absence of fever to any extent. When dry the aspersion was repeated; the shivering diminished at each successive aspersion, until it was entirely allayed. If, on throwing a dog, thus treated, bread, and he will eat it, it is a sign he is cured. Dr. Sully, of Wivelscombe, in a work published some years ago, states, that he dropped water constantly on the wounded part, and that it invariably acted as a preventive. My impression is, that hydropathy is adapted to the cure of this complaint.

CII.—Cholera.

Spasmodic or pestilential cholera first appeared in England in 1831, and in France in 1832; great difference of opinion exists as to its cause, and hardly two practitioners agree as to the best way to effect a cure. Some persons think, as many would get well without medical aid as with it; and this conjecture is supported by what took place on its visitation in Dublin. The numbers attacked were so great, that for the humble class, large tents were erected outside the city, and the medical men were so harassed by their own connexions within it, that the poor were left very much to fate. On comparing notes of the mortality that took place, it was found, that the number of deaths of those who received medical aid, and those who were deprived of it, were about equal. Pages might be employed in enumerating instances related, in which the cholera was cured by cold water, though administered without reference to any hydropathic rules. In 1832, Cholera made great ravages in Silesia, when numbers at Freywaldau and the neighbourhood, fell victims. Priessnitz's patients did not escape, though they avoided its fatal consequences. A friend of mine, who was at Gräfenberg at the time, assures me that in cholera, Priessnitz never lost a case, though seventeen of his patients, and many persons in the neighbourhood, were treated by him. My landlord at Freywaldau, confirmed the last of these statements, and said that his daughter fell a victim, who, he felt persuaded, would have recovered, had she been treated with water instead of drugs.

To ward off this disease, and place the system, if attacked, in the best condition to resist it, we ask the dispassionate reader, are not hydropathic rules in accordance with reason and common sense?

There are three different stages in cholera; the first is that of a common diarrhœa, accompanied with oppression of the chest, anxiety, and collapse of the face; if neglected, it assumes a more serious form, the pulse becomes weak, and there is a difficulty of respiration.

The second stage is ushered in by giddiness, great depression of pulse and of the vital energies, with spasms, accompanied by purging and vomitings.

In the third stage, the patient is suddenly laid prostrate, serous fluid, in large quantities, is discharged from the bowels and stomach, with cramps and spasms, hardly any pulse, and difficult respiration. Under ordinary treatment, this frequently terminates life in a few hours.

To those who have witnessed the wonderful results of the Water-cure treatment in cholic, diarrhœa, &c., it must be evident, that in the primary stages of this malady, the treatment resorted to in those complaints, would be perfectly effectual; and that cholera, in its worst and most fearful form, is to be successfully combated by no other than hydropathic means.

If, after visiting a contagious case, Mr. Priessnitz feels at all uncomfortable, he takes a packing-sheet and tepid-bath.

Asiatic Cholera.—On the first appearance of Cholera symptoms, which are generally those of languor and chilliness, do not wait for a development, but apply most vigorously a rubbing-sheet; then dry the body, and administer a clyster of cold water. In two or three minutes repeat the rubbing-sheet and clyster, wait five minutes and repeat the same a third time. Then a cold sitz-bath, letting two attendants rub the patient with hands dipped in water, particularly on the abdomen, the whole time; water should be drunk whilst in the sitz-bath, until patient vomits; when cramps in the stomach and vomiting have subsided, place a large bandage round the body, and put him to bed well covered up. After sleeping, apply a tepid-bath with friction for some time. If not cured, renew the whole operation.

If, after the sitz-bath, cholera appears on the advance, warm a blanket, and pack the patient as in the sweating process; if he remains therein several hours, and the symptoms do not decrease, renew the whole proceedings, and again try to produce perspiration; when effected, keep it up two or three hours. After this a tepid-bath 62° with friction. The success of the treatment very much depends upon drinking abundantly of water. The bandages used, should be doubled or trebled, and changed often. If patient is unable to stand or sit upright, lay him on a bed, and let several attendants rub him all over with wet hands.

Extract from a letter from Dr. Gibbs to the editor of the "Water-cure Journal."

"You cannot have forgotten the consternation of the profession when this fearful disease invaded us in 1832. Neither can you be ignorant that the faculty, generally, are as ill prepared to contend with it now as they were in former years; but for the information of those who may not be as well acquainted with such matters as you must be, I beg to make an extract from the minutes of the proceedings at a meeting of the Western Medical and Surgical Association, as reported in the *Lancet* of September 19, 1846. In the course of a discussion on the treatment of cholera, Dr. Cahill said, that he 'positively felt a creeping of the skin at the relation of the enormities which had been perpetrated by practitioners upon their patients. When he listened to the recital of practitioners who described the extravagant cases of mercury and of opium which they administered, he could not refrain from fancying that he was witnessing the orgies of so many Indian savages, whilst counting the scalps of their victims. He thought it a pity that the invention of such a system of torture should not experience the fate of the inventor of the brazen bull, and illustrate upon his own person the efficacy of his infernal ingenuity. He believed that in the majority of persons who died of Asiatic cholera, death was the consequence of the treatment rather than of the disease. He had seen above a thousand cases of Asiatic cholera; and in no instance had he seen any benefit from any mode of treatment. On the contrary, he had seen persons die of narcotism, who would have survived if left to the *vis medicatrix naturæ*. He had seen others die of absorption of air through the veins when the saline fluid was ejected; and he knew many who had had the extraordinary luck to escape both the doctor and the disease, yet rendered miserable for the remainder of life by the effects of the immense doses of mercury which had been given to them during the cholera paroxysms. In fact, it was afflicting to contemplate the sufferings which the rash and empirical practice of the profession in the management of this epidemic had created.' The learned gentleman likewise said 'With respect to cholera, since nothing was known of its nature, and no treatment had any influence over it, the best plan was to do as little as possible: give carrara, soda, or pump-water, with a little laudanum, perhaps in the diarrhœal stage, and the patient would not be deprived of the chance which nature had given him.'

"It is to be presumed that the doctor had not seen this disease treated by the Water-cure, under the operation of which, if I am correctly informed, and as I can readily believe, results very different from those, which he witnessed, were obtained. It is stated that more than twenty cases were successfully treated by Priessnitz, and between thirty and forty at Breslau, by a clergyman, whose name I regret that I have forgotten; and it is added that neither practitioner lost a patient by death. The treatment adopted by each of them was nearly the same; the principal difference between them being, that the one employed the sitz-bath, and the other the shallow tepid-bath.

["]If on the appearance of the premonitory symptoms, judicious treatment be promptly adopted, it seems not improbable that the disease may be cut short. Those symptoms may be any combination of the following:— shivering, dizziness, a ringing noise in the ears, a small quick pulse, accelerated respiration, languor, præcordial anxiety, a cold white tongue, nausea, vomiting, severe gripings, and watery diarrhœa. If it be not checked, the disease quickly passes into the second or algid stage; the circulation becomes feeble, the blood is drained of its fluid, the muscles are contracted and cramped, the tongue is colder and whiter, the thirst becomes burning, the lips livid; the features contracted, the extremities shrivelled, and the skin cold, clammy, and discoloured.

"Little is known respecting the nature of this disease; but the most rational opinion seems to be, that it owes its origin to a poison pervading the blood; deranging the balance between the arterial and venous circulation, impairing the nervous energy, and impeding all the functions of the various organs, excepting the secretions from the stomach and bowels; the preternatural excitement of which would seem to indicate an effort of nature to expel the disturbing causes from the system. This opinion obtains additional probability from the fact, which often has been observed, that the more profuse is the diarrhœa, the less fatal is the disease.

"Cholera may suddenly appear without manifesting any, or at least with very slight, premonitory symptoms; especially where the patient is labouring under any serious affection of the brain, lungs, or air-passages, when it will sometimes graft itself on the primary disease, and aggravate all its most various symptoms.

"On the first manifestation of premonitory symptoms, immediate recourse should be had to repeated friction in a wrung-out sheet, as in the earlier stages of fever. This will tend to stimulate the nervous energy, and to maintain or re-establish the balance of circulation between the arterial and venous systems; will counteract the disposition to internal congestion by promoting cuticular circulation; will aid the lungs by freeing the exhalants of the skin, and will forward the elimination of the virus through the same channels.

"But it will not be sufficient merely to attempt to resist the encroachments of the disease; the efforts of nature to expel the cause of it, also claim assistance. To this end cold or tepid water should be freely drunk to facilitate the vomiting, to dilute and weaken the action of the poison, to stimulate the kidneys, and to supply the waste of fluid in the blood. Dr. Rutty, in his synopsis, says, 'It [the drinking of water] has also frequently been found efficacious in stopping violent vomitings and purgings, partly as a diluent, and partly as a bracer to the fibres; and in violent, deplorable choleras, cold water is recommended by the ancients, and at this time is ordered by Spanish physicians with good success, though Celsus orders it warm.'

"Enemata of pure water, tepid or cold, should likewise be freely administered; the quantity administered to an infant at one time should not exceed two ounces; four ounces would be sufficient for a child six years old; eight ounces for a youth of fifteen, and fifteen or sixteen ounces for an adult.

"But the principal process is *long and entire friction,* either in the shallow tepid-bath or in the sitz-bath. The latter seems to deserve the preference, inasmuch as it will more directly and powerfully aid nature in her efforts; its primary action being that of a purgative, while a less body of water will suffice, than could be made to fulfil the same intention in a vessel of the shape and size of the half bath; but, if the sitz-bath be employed, then friction with wet hands should be applied to the extremities. Cold water may be used in the sitz-bath, provided that there is nothing in the previous state of the patient to contra-indicate its use; in which case tepid water must be employed. Tepid water about 70° Fahr. may likewise be employed in the shallow bath, as the body of water therein must be greater than the sitz-bath; but warm applications are never indicated. Vapour-baths have been tried to recall the circulation to the surface, but without effect. On this point, Dr. Daun in his 'Medical Reports on Cholera,' says, 'O'Brien lay on the steam couch for three hours before he expired, in a heat that I am convinced would have raised a lifeless body to a temperature nearly, if not equal, to that of a person in health; but his body preserved an icy coldness to the last.' In this case friction in wrung-out sheets, or in the shallow bath, or perhaps the stimulus of the cold dash, would seem to be indicated.

"Cramps, in the extremities, should be combated with brisk friction, with wet hands to the parts affected. It is often necessary to draw off the urine with a catheter. Before the algid stage sets in, the heating bandage round the body may be very beneficial; but during the algid stage it should be omitted.

"The third stage or that of re-action, is marked by the following, among other symptoms; the pulse becomes fuller and harder, the skin becomes warm, and its livid discoloration disappears; the tongue becomes red and warm, the cramps cease, diarrhœa decreases and stops, and the kidneys begin to act. In this case it is well to encourage moderate diaphoresis in the dry blanket.

"The predisposing causes to cholera are any excess in eating or drinking, the habitual use of alcoholic liquors, unwholesome food, sitting with wet feet, a neglected cold, uncleanliness, impure air, deficient light or ventilation, and violent indulgence of the passions."

CIII.—Colds, Sore Throats, etc.

Influenza.—This complaint which commits such ravages, is always easy of cure.

When a person feels heaviness in the head, sore throat, pain in bowels, and lassitude, he should immediately be put in the packing-sheet until quite hot, then a tepid bath for five or six minutes, and be well rubbed all the time. This treatment to be repeated during the day. Drink plentifully of water, wear a bandage round the waist and throat; if cold and chilly, take two or three rubbing-sheets. To relieve the heaviness of the head, resort to a foot-bath 62° for fifteen minutes. Influenza generally succumbs to this treatment in two or three days.

Sore Throat or Quinzy.—On the slightest symptoms of sore throat, rub it well for five minutes with wet hands two or three times a day; hold cold water constantly in the mouth, and with it gargle the throat, and wear a bandage, this generally prevents the complaint proceeding further; if it does not, more vigorous measures, such as those pointed out for a cold, must be pursued. For Quinzy, the sweating process and tepid-bath twice a day also, or two rubbing-sheets in the intermediate time must be used, a bandage several times doubled and often changed, applied round the throat and waist, and much water drank, gargled, and held in the mouth.

Heaviness after dinner.—Pour a bottle of water on the head, and take head-baths occasionally.

Bronchitis.—In all old affections of the throat a cure is doubtful, it requires the discrimination of Priessnitz to determine which will and which will not be benefited by the Water-cure.

I should say the majority of cases of bronchitis are beyond remedy. At the same time, it cannot be denied that very extraordinary throat affections are cured, especially when they arise from secondary symptoms.

Palpitation of the Heart, stitches in the side, etc.—A young lady felt violent palpitation of the heart, and numbness of the whole side of the body. Three-rubbing sheets and a foot-bath with friction, allayed the palpitation, then a body *umschlag* was applied. Next night the same symptoms returned, and were combated in the like manner, afterwards the patient was treated with packing-sheets, tepid-bath, foot-bath, and douche. Whenever any obstructions of this nature occur, it is always safe to resort to rubbing-sheets two or three times a day.

Erysipelas.—This disease is an effort of nature to relieve itself by the skin; the packing-sheet process in this case is resorted to, followed by a rubbing-sheet or tepid-bath: when the head is overcharged, sometimes the body is placed in a packing-sheet (previously put into tepid water instead of cold) from the arm-pits to the knees, and then a tepid-bath or a bath with very little water in it. Much water should be drunk, and bandages applied to parts affected.

To refresh and invigorate.—A gentleman with no decided complaint, but generally feeling a degree of languor, and want of nervous energy was ordered, a rubbing-sheet in the morning and afternoon, and a sitz-bath in the middle of the day, followed by much exercise.

Another party felt somewhat below his usual standard of health and activity. For years there had been an accumulation of matter in his nose, from which at times there was a free discharge. Priessnitz said it was a sort of safety valve, and had better not be stopped: the patient derived great advantage from pursuing the following treatment for six weeks:—

In the morning, a packing-sheet for twenty minutes, then changed for another for fifteen minutes; this was followed, first by tepid, and afterwards by cold bath; at noon, a rubbing-sheet and sitz-bath for fifteen minutes; head-bath three minutes each side, making in all nine minutes; in the afternoon, rubbing-sheet, sitz and head-bath.

CIV.—CANCER, ETC.

When taken in the commencement, this disease is generally curable; later, a cure admits of doubt.

Princess Esterhazy, who was so long in England, consulted all the leading medical men in Vienna for a cancer in the breast: they could afford her no relief. She went to Gräfenberg and was perfectly cured in seven months. Six years afterwards, one of the family informed me she still continued in perfect health.

A neighbour of Priessnitz had a cancer in his hip; he advised him not to allow of an operation, as it would grow again. The man disregarded this advice, it did grow again, and his life paid the forfeit. A general treatment is required for this complaint.

Our opinion that water, even without Priessnitz's valuable modes of applying it, is the best remedy—is supported by Dr. Abernethy, who, in his book entitled "Surgical Observations", mentions a case of a lady (page 200), who had gone up to town for the removal of a diseased breast, who was cured without amputation, the only local application being linen moistened with water. Dr. Abernethy applied water poultices also for glandular swellings, which had the effect of removing the swelling without suppuration—*see pages* 189 and 192. I know a French lady who cured herself of a hard swelling on the breast: she took a rubbing-sheet every morning, a sitz-bath at mid-day, drank ten tumblers of water daily, and wore a wet bandage, with a dry one over it, on the breast always, until the hardness was removed.

A case of White Swelling.—A letter from Dr. Gibbs to the Editor of the Water-cure Journal.

"My dear Sir, "*March, 17th, 1848.*

"I have heard even friends of the Water-cure express doubts of its efficacy in the treatment of white swelling. For the benefit of such unbelievers I transcribe the case at foot, from a letter which I received from the mother of the youthful patient.

"The enemies of the system frequently assert that it cures only imaginary diseases; how many would rejoice if it could be proved that white swelling properly came under this category!

"From the details of this case, it appears that, by the advice of Priessnitz, an operation was performed by the late very eminent surgeon, Dieffenbach; and this affords occasion to observe, that Dieffenbach several times remarked, that patients sent to him from Water-cure establishments were in a healthier condition for the knife than others, and more speedily recovered from the effects of an operation.

"'Until the age of four years my daughter was perfectly healthy, when, at the commencement of winter, she was attacked by cough and wheezing on her chest, which gave the idea that her lungs were affected. Leeches were applied, and medicine given with little effect. She continued to look very ill, and became extremely peevish and inactive. In the spring she was suddenly seized by a pain in her left knee, which rendered her quite lame. The complaint was pronounced to be white swelling. One of our first surgeons assured me the attack was of a most acute nature, the joint of the knee being considerably enlarged, and the suffering very great. By steam-baths and leeching the inflammation was in some degree subdued, and mercury was used in various ways, internally, and externally. In a week or ten days the violent pain subsided, but she could not bear the limb to be moved in the slightest manner. In that state the child continued for eighteen months, during which she had three acute attacks similar to the first, which were got under in the same manner, after each attack the limb became more contracted, and the constitution was evidently sinking, although wine, porter, and fresh meat, etc. etc., were allowed, in order to keep up her strength, but they did not succeed. She was at the sea-side for the benefit of the bathing, which appeared to strengthen her more than anything else, when I learned something of the water system from Captain Claridge's book, and subsequently from himself. At first, I must confess, I was rather startled at the idea of trying such an experiment on my child, but, as every thing else had failed, I made up my mind to go to Gräfenberg and put her into the hands of Mr. Priessnitz. In the beginning of September he commenced with her, giving her at first two packings up and a tepid bath, and one knee-bath during the day, and compresses on the knee and body. He desired that she should have crutches, and try to move about as much as she could without hurting herself. She continued the same treatment during the ensuing winter, during which she had a constant rash on her entire leg, and subsequently several gatherings on and round the knee, none on any other part of her body. In the spring she commenced the cold bath after the packing up, and the douche bath. Her strength increased rapidly, her looks became quite healthy, and her appetite excellent. The appearance of the knee was very variable until the end of the summer, when it diminished considerably in size, and she could bear to have it moved without any annoyance; but about Christmas it became suddenly nearly as bad as ever it had been. All cure was then stopped, except one packing up and tepid bath, and the knee compresses were changed every quarter of an hour. The inflammation and pain were soon got under, but she continued the slight cure until the spring, when she commenced the packing up and cold bathing twice a day—douche-bath twice, and knee-bath twice, with rubbing with the wet hand, and compresses changed after every operation. During this summer she made a wonderful improvement, and the limb became so strong that she could bear to have it pulled so as to drag her about by it. Mr. Priessnitz said he thought the child was now quite free from *all disease*, and that I might have an operation performed to straighten the limb, in which opinion several English medical men quite agreed with him. I then took her to Berlin, having been two years at Gräfenberg; the leg was made quite straight by Dr. Dieffenbach, and since then the child enjoys perfect health, being quite strong on her limbs, though still somewhat lame. She continues the use of the cold bath and douche every day. It is generally thought that she will outgrow the lameness. I forgot to mention that from the time the knee was attacked, the chest and cough quite recovered.'"

Swallowing Glass.—A cure effected in the house of the Princess Sophia, by her priest, the Rev. Mr. Klose:—

June 1st, 1843.

A married woman, 26 years of age, in eating, swallowed a piece of glass, which stuck in her throat; after many unavailing efforts, either to force it up or down, she sent for a surgeon, who gave her an emetic, which also proved unavailing; then he tried to extract it with instruments, and applied a number of leeches to the throat, *to no effect*. The second day, the surgeon declared he could do no more, and she was attacked with inflammatory fever. As a *dernier ressort*, Mr. Klose determined on trying hydropathy.

She was enveloped and kept in the wet sheet, with bandages round the throat, day and night, both being changed as soon as they became warm.

At the beginning of this treatment, the invalid was unable to swallow even a drop of water, could scarcely breathe, and a horrid smell came from the mouth. Her medical attendant said that mortification had set in, and gave it as his opinion, that she could not live through the next day.

Third and fourth days, the same treatment was continued, with the addition of three enemas, which operated slightly. The packing-sheet, instead of being changed, was wetted with a sponge: moving the body occasioned pain. She threw up a great deal of phlegm and matter, which stank so horribly, that no person could remain near her bed-side.

Fifth day.—Vomiting increased, also the heat of the whole body; the increase of heat rendered it necessary (notwithstanding the pain she felt on being moved) to administer a tepid-bath 18°. Whilst in the bath, her head, throat, and chest, were frequently wetted with cold water, and the abdomen and feet were well rubbed. This bath afforded her great relief, and whilst in it, she threw up much matter with ease and without coughing. She remained in the bath thirty-five minutes, the same temperature of the water being maintained throughout. At the expiration of this time, the body was considerably cooled, but the pulse was still very high; for which reason, recourse was again had to the packing-sheet, which produced a regularity of the pulse. She was now enabled to swallow the first drop of water.

Sixth day.—Mortification pronounced to be subdued, but as she could not take anything in the way of nourishment, four injections of milk were administered, and when fever returned, water injections instead of milk were given.

Seventh day.—Besides the former treatment, a tepid-bath was administered, with the same effect as on the fifth day, viz. much vomiting and decrease of cough.

Eighth day.—Patient much better, treatment in consequence changed, only large bandages being applied to the chest, throat, and neck, and in the afternoon she could swallow some cold thin soup.

Ninth day.—Heat and fever returned, large quantities of matter vomited, and inflammation of windpipe. Treatment changed back again to packing-sheet and bandage and one tepid-bath.

Tenth, Eleventh, and Twelfth days, same treatment.

Thirteenth day.—Fever ceased, vomiting diminished, and patient able to swallow some milk and water.

Fourteenth and Fifteenth days.—Great improvement, could eat a little apple sauce.

Sixteenth day.—Some fever, but she could swallow some spoonfuls of milk without coughing.

Seventeenth day.—After a tolerably quiet night, there was found in the bed a piece of glass, which must have been thrown up by coughing.

Eighteenth, Nineteenth, Twentieth, and Twenty-first days.—Great improvement, and diminution of vomiting, also of bad smell. She drank, and ate some light food very slowly, but without coughing.

Twenty-second day to 8th July.—Every day improvement, recovering strength, and walking a little in the garden.

9th July.—Went to church.

10th.—Resumed her occupations, quite well, except when working she suffered some slight pain, which ceased when she rested.

Mr. Wright's case.—(Extract from a letter)—"Diseased lungs, breathing organs generally impaired, chest, formerly full and prominent, fallen in, breathing difficult, sleep disturbed, dry cough, sometimes painful, for more than a year; a short walk caused perspiration, 46 years old, formerly robust, healthy, and strong.

"Cold water my only beverage for fifteen years, no alcohols.

"Three years ago began flannels, fur muffles round neck. Used every possible precaution to keep the fresh air from throat, chest, body, and lungs.

"Habituated to cold ablutions, it never occurred to me, that if the body could stand these ablutions, no ill consequences could result from admitting the air freely to it.

"Began hydropathic treatment at Gräfenberg, 10th January, 1843, thermometer at zero. At once abandoned all flannels, and superfluous covering. Linen shirts substituted for cotton ones.

"Treatment:—two packing-sheets, followed by tepid-bath, a day; at eleven o'clock sitz-bath. Waist bandages always. Drank ten tumblers of water before breakfast. Hail, rain, or snow, always walked before breakfast; soon commenced the douche and two rubbing-sheets of an afternoon, instead of the packing-sheets.

"From the first, found the treatment, the exercise and pure air, exceedingly stimulating.

"Neck, throat, and chest, exposed in all weathers. In three months a rash was produced; appetite voracious, breathing improved, cough ceased.

"About 1st April, joints, especially knees, began to grow stiff, sore, and weak—pain in walking, and difficulty of straightening knees after sitting.

Low and gloomy in spirits, and altogether disheartened; told by people around it was a good sign; the treatment was taking effect, and so indeed I found it, affecting body and soul.

"Whole body became very sensitive to the touch of cold water; it seemed as if the nerves were laid bare; in fact, had a perfect horror of the treatment, which became more intolerable as the season advanced and became damp. Damp weather of April worse than the cold of January and February. Now became afflicted with throbbing pains in teeth, jaws, and face, attended with sickness, for which I rubbed the back of my head, neck, and face with cold water, and also my knees frequently.

"This," says Mr. Wright, "was the crisis of my misery. The most enthusiastic hydropathist could not have wished me more wretched than I was. It appears to me, the only way to a cold water heaven, is through a cold water purgatory. I was frequently congratulated on my sufferings, as one making a speedy and radical cure.

"Latter end of April, boils made their appearance on arms, hands, fingers, and other parts of the body. All came to a head, and healed during the month of May, and more succeeded them.

"Continued treatment vigorously, exposing myself to atmospheric changes as much as possible. I now feel, that *all disease of my lungs is removed. My chest has resumed its natural fulness, my cough is entirely* gone, and my voice is as strong and as deep-toned as it ever was. Altogether my physical nature has experienced a great renovation. I can now walk six or eight miles before breakfast without fatigue. I have walked, on an average, about ten miles a-day since at Gräfenberg. What of life, of usefulness, of health and comfort that remains to me in this world, I owe to the Water-cure under Providence, and to the kind friends who, much against my will, compelled me to come to Gräfenberg. Nothing surprised me so much, as the perfect safety with which I cast off my warm comfortable flannels, mufflers, neckcloth, hat, etc. Inflamed lungs, and an increase of my cough, were the least that I expected; but I was most agreeably disappointed, for although frequently wet through, and my neck, chest, and the hair of my head (as I always went bare-headed) constantly covered with snow, my lungs have always escaped, nor have I had a cold, that a packing-sheet, or one night's bandage has not removed. I frequently, on arriving at my room drenched with rain, wet, and fatigued, took a rubbing-sheet, which prevented all evil consequences, and invigorated me.

"From what I have experienced and seen in others, I can never again fear cold, influenza, or fevers of any kind, as I feel sufficient confidence to treat myself. The most malignant acute diseases are here speedily and easily subdued, and that by a remedy which leaves no sting behind, whilst drugs often leave an enemy in the system more difficult to expel, than *that* they were intended to eject.

"It is surprising what confidence all exhibit in the cure and its practitioners. We have just had a case of small-pox, of the most malignant kind. Persons passed through the passage into which the patient's room opened all day long. The same bath-servant that attended him attended other patients. The latter went into his room constantly to see him. His wife attended him, and yet no one thought of taking the disease; or if he did, had any fear of it, knowing from what we had previously witnessed, that it was entirely under the control of this treatment.

"The patient was confined to his room fourteen days, the disease broke out from head to foot.

"After the fourteen days, he walked out amongst the other patients, and the wonder is, that nearly every trace of disease is passing from his face.

"Treatment.—Packing-sheets, tepid-bath, rubbing-sheets and fresh air were the only remedies."

"June 20th.

"Before closing, I wish to add, I suffered much from tooth-ache and pain in my jaws. Priessnitz ordered me to rub the back of my head and down my neck *often* and *long*. From the first application I found relief, after fourteen or fifteen minutes rubbing. The pain would leave for hours and then return; soon the pain returned at longer intervals, until it ceased altogether.

"The theory of this mode of curing tooth-ache, is based upon true philosophical principles. Who does not know, that all the nerves of the teeth centre in the back of the head? It is evident then, that by rubbing there, the pain will be drawn from the teeth.

"I have now been three months out of the treatment, only continuing the bath and rubbing-sheet; neither of which shall I ever abandon, as I consider them luxuries, and preventives of disease. I would rather be deprived of one of my daily meals, than of either of them. I am now well, and about to return to the field of my labours.

"Whoever is ill and not passed recovery, may, I believe, find health by the treatment administered by Priessnitz, provided he is willing to labour for it, but if any one expects to find it whilst wrapped up in flannels, lounging in easy chairs or on sofas, in confined rooms, or without great self-denial, personal activity and exertion, he will, most certainly, be disappointed.

"HENRY C. WRIGHT,
"Philadelphia, U. S.
"June 21st, 1844."

"*To Jno. Gibbs, Esq.*"

The Countess of Jennison's case.—The Countess, who had only been married seven weeks, went to visit the Princess Tour and Taseis, when she joined in skating, dancing, and playing at various games. On her return home, she was seized with a violent head-ache, when a blister was administered to the back of her neck. The pain continuing, a blister was applied to the chest, and subsequently to other parts, all without avail. Several doctors were consulted, whose measures weakened her nerves. A severe nervous fever ensued, which deprived her entirely of the use of her limbs. After seven months' extreme suffering, and the speculative operations of various medical men, the case was declared a hopeless one.

She made her will, received the sacrament, and was at times quite unconscious of what was passing around. Her debility may be judged of by the fact that she could neither move joint nor limb, nor even close her mouth or eyes. She was mere skin and bones, and her knuckles became black.

Her husband, as a *dernier ressort,* went to Gräfenberg to consult Priessnitz, the result of which was, Mrs. Browne, a bath-woman, going to Brünn to bring the Countess to Gräfenberg, Priessnitz persisting in it, that by management she could be brought. When Mrs. Browne stated her intention to the M.D.'s in attendance, nothing could exceed their astonishment. The first thing this bath-woman did, preparatory to the journey, was to wash the body with tepid water, and it is heart-rending to hear her account of the manner in which tow had been allowed to fix itself in the hips, elbows, and other parts exposed to pressure; however, little by little she succeeded in cleansing the body of all these medical applications. She then ordered an upholsterer to make a soft, narrow, mattress, with a number of tapes attached to it, and the Count arranged the carriage so that the body might be extended in it.

The next morning, all being ready, Mrs. Browne bound up the arms, the legs, and the whole of the body, in a number of wet bandages, with dry ones over them, by this means there was more pliancy to the whole frame than if it had been confined in one sheet, and it was much easier to exchange the different bandages when they became dry *en route*.

The Countess was now fixed on the mattrass by means of the tapes, and then placed into the carriage: in this manner she proceeded, night and day, stopping occasionally to change the bandages. Had these bandages become dry, they would not have been endurable. In this way the patient arrived at the Hygeian Temple.

It would be impossible to give a detailed account of the Countess's treatment during the time she was attaining to convalescence. As a general outline, it may be stated, that when first brought to Gräfenberg, she was constantly kept in a packing-sheet from the arm-pits downwards. Her feet were kept in water, with but slight intervals, day and night for months; even when somewhat better, and able to go out in a carriage, her feet were in cold water. Priessnitz did not wish this, but her feet burned so dreadfully when out of water, that there was no alternative. During the first four months of the treatment, enemas were administered, nature being too weak to assist itself. When she had gained a little strength, her hands were put on the table and pushed on a few inches by her attendant, and the same with her feet. She could not move them herself. After four months she was strong enough for the douche and cold-bath.

The packing-sheets were changed when dry—at times in fever they were hot in ten minutes, at other times two packing-sheets a day were sufficient.

At the end of forty-nine weeks she left strong and healthy, able to walk without sticks, and was three months advanced in pregnancy.

1845.

Four years after I met the Countess again, at Gräfenberg, and was astonished to behold her such a fine, fat, healthy woman. Since being cured she has had three children, one died almost immediately after its birth, the second is a fine child, and for her accouchement of the third, she came to place herself under the care of Priessnitz. She did remarkably well, and left Gräfenberg in perfect health.

I consider this one of the most wonderful cures effected by Priessnitz. Those who saw the complete *anatomie vivante*, which she was, declared that nothing but a miracle could save her from her early tomb.

HYDROPATHY FOR ANIMALS.

The unspeakable utility of the horse to man in all conditions of life, civilised and uncivilised, has naturally led scientific and professional individuals to devote much anxious consideration to the physiology of the animal, and to the determination of the means of healing the diseases which horse-flesh "is heir to." Buffon placed the horse next to man in the order of creation; and certainly if the anatomical structure of the equine species be alone regarded, an argument is provided in favor of the consecration of thought and intelligence to the establishment of curative remedies for its disorders. But the service which the noble animal has rendered in all ages and countries where the breed is known—his docility, instinct, patience, and courage, have entitled him to the advantages of human intelligence upon the high ground of gratitude; and, accordingly, for many years past, the veterinary art has been pursued with remarkable zeal and earnestness; the loftiest minds not conceiving the study and practice thereof below their attention. If, however, the attainment of perfection in the faculty of curing the bodily ailments of man is a work of tardy progress, how much slower must be the advancement of a science of posterior introduction? It was but in the last century that the circulation of the blood was discovered, and vaccination introduced; it is only within the last six or seven years that the vast utility of hydropathy has come to be appreciated. There is now, however, less excuse for dilatory improvement in veterinary practice than there was when the alleviation of human suffering was in its infancy. The physiology and pathology of the quadruped being understood, the value of the immediate adoption of the remedies applicable to man is at once determinable by anatomical analogy. Hence the introduction of new systems of treatment has been almost simultaneous, and in very many instances the results have been correspondingly fortunate. Hydropathy is a very remarkable case in point, and the following pages will illustrate its value.

Priessnitz's precepts recommend themselves as much to the veterinary surgeon as to the medical practitioner; the success of his treatment of the diseased animal being, perhaps, even more easy and certain than of man.

To understand this it will suffice to compare the habits and mode of living of each. A further investigation will account for the general health of untamed animals, and the host of maladies that result from civilisation. On one side all is nature, on the other all is artificial.

As the treatment of the horse or cow at Gräfenberg is not of very frequent occurrence, Priessnitz has not laid down any positive rules for the manipulation; that must therefore depend upon the ingenuity, observation, and experience, of the practitioner.

If, for instance, a horse or cow is attacked with fever, cholic, etc., reference should be made to the treatment of man affected with such complaints. All that has been said on the subject of drugs, the lancet, cold ablutions, and the importance of the skin applies equally to all animals.

How can we expect to cure horses with poisons?

How get them into condition, by depriving them of their blood?

A gentleman of high standing in society, and well known in the sporting world, having, some years since, derived great advantage from the Water-cure, determined on trying its effects upon animals, by becoming his own veterinary surgeon; the consequence is, that for five or six years he has not spent one shilling upon drugs of any kind. On being applied to for his opinion as to the effect of the treatment upon horses, he favored the author with a letter of which the following is an extract:

"With respect to the treatment of horses, my groom can give no information, excepting indeed, that he can verify the good effect of the treatment insisted upon by myself; and such is his prejudice (exactly similar to that of the Medical Profession) that he would, I am sure, revert to his former practices if he dared. But I can most safely affirm that the effect of the Hydro-therapeutic Treatment of Horses, is most wonderful. I have, with coach horses and hacks, say forty horses. I never allow of any bleeding or physic. When the hunters are to be prepared for the season, two or three of a day are whisped over with cold water, a linen cloth of fifteen or sixteen yards in length, dipped in cold water and well wrung out, is then lapped round from their heads to their tails, covered over with rugs, and bound pretty close by surcingles: thus they remain for an hour or so, when they are again rubbed over with cold water, followed by rubbing with dry cloth or whisps quite dry, and then sent out to exercise for twenty-five minutes, or half an hour. This treatment is continued twice or thrice a week, for *at least* half a dozen times; and I'll venture to say that nobody's horses can look, or go better; and they never ail. I will just relate one fact. I bought a horse for Mrs. —— seven or eight years ago, a most excellent lady's horse, but he coughed so badly (always) three or four years since, that we thought she would be obliged to give him up, he has been treated as above for two years; I rode him a gallop a few days ago, when he had not a symptom of cough. Many dealers have been through my stable:—Smart, Elmore, etc. etc., and they have all adopted my plan of bandaging the legs of their horses, which I do for two days after a day's work; and as Elmore said last spring, they looked 'as if they were going to begin a season instead of ending one,' so clear were their legs.

"If a new horse (which is often the case) comes down by railroad, he generally gets a sore throat and cold, this, I need not tell you, is soon got rid of, as above."—*May 4, 1848.*

The following extract is from a letter to the author—written by a gentleman whose health has been re-established by the Water-cure; who, during the last forty years, has been the possessor of hundreds of horses, and is said to be one of the best judges of a horse in England.

"I will not defer answering your interesting letter, although I know not that I can write anything to be of much use to you. The manner in which I have treated my horses for the last thirty years is as follows:—If it is in my power I always bring a horse in cool, my groom first puts a common watering bridle on, takes one girth off, and slackens the other, the reason why I do not remove the saddle immediately is, because the back becomes tender; the horse is then taken into the pond, the boy holding up his own legs, the higher the water gets towards the back the better; that is, let the animal go as deep into water as he can, not to swim; this takes two or three minutes, then two men take scrapers, and with these press out the dripping water, after this, with straw whisps, the animal is washed for about ten minutes, he is then covered up with two blankets, and his legs bandaged; the ears are now well rubbed and pulled until dry: this is all I do to a horse. He does not break out into cold perspirations during the night, and next morning he is perfectly clean. By putting your hands under the blankets when he is done up for the night, you will find a genial warmth pervading the whole body. Blood horses, however fatigued, are usually very sensitive to the brush and whisp, consequently cleaning tires them still more, which causes them almost always to break out into cold sweats. The ventilation which ought to be at the top of the stable, must be good, otherwise the system works ill. Owing to the unusual good health that I have had in my stable, I was led to think most seriously of applying water in a similar way to the human subject, so that after reading your book, I became at once a confirmed Hydropathist. Many people will say, my system was that pursued in the post-horse stables; but the contrary is the fact. The post horse was washed, and his heels clipped close, and left to dry without friction, evaporation was great, grease and other maladies attacked the animal. I know a coach master who saved £400 per annum by giving up washing upon this old plan. You have now got the result of my experience. I have had fewer roarers than most men for the number of horses in my possession, in fact, only two, one of these went so, when lent and out of my stable. The loss in valuable horses from roaring is enormous. I think a friend of mine lost £700 in one season from roarers, I have the confidence to think that had he pursued the Water-system all his horses would have been saved. Be assured, water is as applicable to the animal as the human subject—fever is the bane of the one as much as the other, and water is the antidote. Why are cart-horses so much healthier than higher fed horses? simply because the former live much more after nature than the other. A cart-horse goes to a pond and drinks what he likes, not so with the blood horse, he must only have a certain quantity, and this at stated periods; this I conceive to be wrong, and have in consequence for the last six years always kept buckets of water in the horses' boxes, so that they might drink when they liked. My friends have often said, 'But you do not allow them thus to drink when going to hunt?' 'Certainly' was my reply: if the animal always has access to water, he never distends his stomach, and by constantly sipping, fever is kept down. We do all we can to encourage fever, and then have recourse to strong drastics and bleeding! Constant water cools the animal, and the gentle sweats, which the blankets produce, operate as safety valves."—*January 5, 1848.*

When in Ireland, visiting the far-famed dairy farm of Mr. Jefferies, in the neighbourhood of Cork, I was informed by the bailiff, that out of every seven cows attacked with an epidemic which raged at that time, on an average five had died, and that the loss on that estate had not been less than 2000*l*. On my suggesting hydropathic treatment, the bailiff said that some time ago a traveller by that means had cured him of rheumatism; this determined him on trying it upon the cows: success crowned his efforts; instead of losing five out of seven, he saved seven out of nine; this treatment, however, at once so novel and so troublesome, he found extremely difficult to prosecute, servants could not be induced to use the necessary friction, or endure the toil which a number of sick animals entail: this, together with the discouragement and ridicule thrown upon his proceedings by the veterinary surgeon, caused him to desist. The following is a letter which I subsequently read from the bailiff—

"Dear Sir—I am most anxious to communicate with you as to the efficacy of the cold-water cure, when applied to cattle affected with the late epidemic.

"About six months ago, I had it tried on nine head of horned cattle; seven out of the nine recovered, and are now doing well. I feel quite confident that, if the cure be generally known, and properly applied, much may be done in the recovering of diseased cattle.

"I am, Dear Sir, your obedient servant,
["]THOMAS B. MARTIN.

["]*July 14, 1843.*["]

It is possible that the omission of any reference to the mortality under the old treatment, as stated verbally to me, may have arisen from motives of delicacy towards those who recommended a perseverance in that treatment.

It would be easy to multiply instances of the effect of the application of the cold-water cure, but as the limits to which the author intends to confine himself, at present preclude their accumulation, he must be content with those proofs of its efficacy already cited, and proceed to the subject of *treatment*.

An opinion is held by many inexperienced persons that disease in a horse is a perpetual disqualification; that the physical evil is irradicable, destroying the animal's title to a future warranty, and rendering him only fit for the paddock or the knacker's yard. Such notions are as great an outrage upon the usefulness of veterinarianism as they are contradictory to all experience. The late Sir Astley Cooper, one of the most eminent surgeons that ever dignified the profession by his talents, was said to have taken a peculiar pleasure in purchasing horses which their owners had condemned, and applying himself to the cure of such maladies as they might be afflicted with, then putting them into condition and selling them. He never, for many years before his demise, gave more than seven pounds for a horse, and has been known to sell them afterwards for considerable sums. When the horse is well-bred, and his wind is unimpaired, however reduced he may be, and suffering from enlarged joints and tender feet, he is still susceptible of cure; and no system is so conducive to this end as the hydropathic process. Indeed, the writer of these pages is quite satisfied that an Establishment devoted entirely to the invigoration of worn-down animals, and the complete cure of the diseased, would demonstrate the utility of hydropathy, and prove a most lucrative undertaking.

Without further preamble we proceed to details.

Ventilation.—The introduction of fresh air, day and night, into stables, is of primary importance. Stables should be lofty, and ventilated from the top.

Many years ago, Mr. Horne, the coach-proprietor of Charing Cross, lost nearly half his horses from glanders. He called in a new veterinary surgeon, who instantly broke most of the windows in the close fœtid stable. "If," said he, "the stable is cold, cover the horses better, but let them have fresh air." By this means the stable was rendered wholesome, and the horses that were afterwards put into it continued healthy. All horses would be the better for standing in water occasionally. All hunting establishments should have a box with a clay floor, into which water could be introduced, so that a horse might have a foot bath every day, especially when the feet are hard and dry.

Food and Exercise.—The arguments made use of against highly nutritive food, and the necessity for exposure to cold and exercise for man apply with equal cogency to animals.

Mr. Newman, the postmaster in Regent-street, has no racks in his stable; but his horses, at stated periods, eat chaff and oats mixed together: he gives them no hay. This method of feeding horses is found economical and healthy. A friend of mine feeds all his farm horses as he does his oxen and pigs, upon Indian corn, oil cake, chaff, and bruised beans boiled up together. He never gives them any oats, and no horses in the kingdom look in finer condition.

Sudorific Process.—This is the same for horses as for men; and is often sufficient to effect a cure, as the greatest part of the diseases of horses proceed from suppressed perspiration. In a general way packing-sheets and consequent ablutions will effect all that may be necessary to cure a horse or a cow of an acute attack, but instances as in man, may occur, when sweating would be desirable.

To produce perspiration in a horse the same objection to the use of hot-air or vapour baths, exists as in the treatment or man; but as the animal's skin and nervous system is less excitable, it does not apply to the same extent.

To sweat a horse, that is to bring out of his system a certain amount of caloric. Throw many pails of water over him, let his body be rubbed with wet whisps for from five to twenty minutes, and then rubbed dry. Next envelope him from head to foot in blankets, and over them throw a Macintosh cover. This might be made to be put on with very little trouble. After the horse has perspired, for an hour or two he must have a cold bath or undergo the process of water being thrown over him, of being wet, whisped, and dried as before. And the whole should be renewed a second time during the day. Or varied by the packing sheet.

External use of Cold Water.—Friction with coarse wet cloths or whisps, packing-sheets, sweating, entire-baths, hip-baths, foot-baths, douche-baths, and bandages, constitute all the external treatment requisite for a horse. Friction by rubbing the body of the animal for some hours with coarse cloths, and whisps of wetted straw, is an operation of great efficacy in bringing out stagnant humours, reanimating half paralysed limbs, and in strengthening the joints. The douche, where no other can be had, is applied by means of a fire-engine. The baths have the property of giving a tone to the skin and the nerves. The bandages for the horse are the same as those used for man; they are of two sorts, heating and cooling.

Internal use of Cold Water.—There are two ways of applying cold water internally, viz.: drinks and injections into the cavities; but ablutions long continued and often repeated form the most important part of the treatment.

The Strangles.—This disease is cured by the wet sheet packing, or the sudorific process, cold-ablution bandages and exercise.

It is much better, by either of these processes, to draw the humours to the skin, which they undoubtedly will, than to throw them on the lungs, whence they escape by the nostrils, a means of evacuation chosen by nature. The natural course being impeded, open the pores of the cutaneous organs, and the running at the nostrils will cease.

Foundering of horses.—Friction, the wet-sheet or sudorific process, the douche and foot-baths, are here brought into requisition.

The Staggers.—Bleeding procures a temporary relief, but does not remove the cause of this complaint, which arises from a stoppage of perspiration, and consequent inertness of the skin. The humours which ought to be eliminated by perspiration mix with and thicken the blood; this causes a general stagnation which frequently affects the brain. This, it is conceived, must be a solution of this malady, because in the beginning one single friction, powerfully applied, affords immediate relief.

In severe cases, the animal should be subjected to the sweating process, and cold ablution. The animal's head should be wetted every hour with cold water, and green food prescribed as a diet. The douche in these cases is of the greatest utility.

Weakness of the Limbs, and Sprains.—These affections are generally successfully treated by constant friction with cold water. This rubbing subdues the heat; bandages should be continually worn. The weakness of the hips and loins soon disappears under this treatment; the douche in these cases is highly beneficial.

Broken Knees.—Let the part be carefully washed, then bandages applied *above*, and *below*, and *upon* the part affected, and kept continually wet as long as inflammation continues. After which, use wet bandages, covered with dry ones, until the part is healed.

External Inflammation and Wounds.—After having well cleaned the sore, it should be covered with a heating-bandage; and if the inflammation is severe, and the heat great, the bandage should be frequently renewed. The animal should take a bath, but without wetting the wound.

External inflammation proceeds from two causes; first, the tightness of the saddle, which wounds the flesh; secondly, from the blows which the horse receives. As soon as you perceive that the horse has been hurt by the saddle, take it off, and having rubbed him well dry, place upon the wound a heating-bandage, firmly tied on, and let it be frequently renewed; but always before renewing the bandage, clean the part affected with cold water; the parts near the wound must be treated in the same manner. This bandage and friction are useful in cases of throat obstructions; the bandage must be changed as often as it becomes hot. Before it becomes quite dry, it should be renewed, taking care each time to rub well the parts affected, which renders them, when exposed, less sensitive. This gives elasticity to the wound.

Tender Feet.—All horses should stand upon clay, bricks, or stones; not upon straw, as it heats the feet too much. For corns or tender feet, foot-baths for an hour or two, two or three times a day are resorted to; and bandages should be worn from the fetlock to the knee-joints, to draw the heat from the feet. A friend of the author's, travelling on the Continent, tried this on a mare which became lame: it succeeded admirably.

Cholic.—Apply one or two clysters of cold water; wet the body, and rub the animal well for an hour with wet whisps, and then put round the body a sheet wetted and doubled several times, covered with a dry blanket. If the first operation is not sufficient, resort to the packing process, and afterwards the rubbing. This system persevered in, the cholic is sure to give way.

Lock-Jaw.—Friction, the douche, and perspiration, are the remedies resorted to. During the intervals of their application, cold bandages should be applied.

The irritation of the skin counteracts the lock-jaw. The efficiency of cold water in this complaint has been known in England for years. An article, some time ago, appeared in the Chelmsford paper, stating that the possessor of a valuable horse, which had been seized with lock-jaw, after trying all other means in vain, threw from the loft, upon the animal, a hogshead or more of water, and then had him covered up in blankets. This brought on perspiration, and a cure was the result. An acquaintance of the author's, in Gloucester[s]hire, who treated a horse in a similar way, was equally successful.

Fever and Inflammation.—For the treatment of all fevers and inflammations the reader is referred to the method prescribed for human beings in similar cases.

For a horse in a high state of inflammation, Priessnitz prescribed his being put into a river for five minutes, then taken out, rubbed dry, for five minutes, then put again into the water and again rubbed, a process renewed until the inflammation had completely subsided. Sometimes this is effected in a short time; at others, it requires constant application for seven or eight hours. Perseverance in this treatment is certain of effecting a cure.

In an ordinary case of fever, resort to the wet-sheet packing; if necessary, change the sheet often, then administer a cold bath or affusion; repeat the operation twice a-day.

In all cases of inflammation or fever, if the body is confined, it is necessary to resort to clysters.

Want of appetite.—If frictions with wisps of straw upon a wet surface repeated three times a day do not produce appetite, the wet-sheet packing followed by ablutions and bandages must be resorted to.

To refresh and invigorate a horse.—Let him be well rubbed with coarse wet cloths or whisps of hay for an hour or two twice a day, then walked about until dry: a foot bath twice a-day for an hour each time, and the loins and legs bandaged.

If the skin of the animal is dry and contracted, use the packing sheet twice a day followed by cold-bath, or throw several pails of water over the body, use friction until the skin is dry, then bandage round the body.

If horses are allowed to be out at grass, they ought, nevertheless, to undergo the operations. With certain exceptions it would be better to keep horses up and send them out to exercise at stated times.

After every operation animals ought to be led about a little.

Murrain amongst cattle.—On the first symptom of the disease, such as the coat starting, the animal is to be subjected to the treatment until shivering is produced, and until shivering has ceased, or at least greatly decreased.

This will require, generally, one, two, or three hours. The animal should stand in a cold bath, that is, a pond or river, and water must be continually thrown over the whole body.

During the whole operation, the body and legs of the animal must be well rubbed with the hand, or with a coarse cloth or whisp (that is, whilst in the bath).

It will require two men to do this properly. Should the water be too deep for the men and sufficiently deep to cover the back, the animal must remain five minutes in the water, be then taken out and well rubbed for five minutes, and so continued till the shivering described above is produced.

Should shivering *not* be produced the case is hopeless.

On coming out of the bath, rub the animal for five minutes, then give him half an hour's walking exercise, with a warm rug as a covering.

The bath is to be repeated twice a-day. After exercise a large piece of coarse cloth wetted with cold water is to be placed over the body and chest, this wet linen is to be covered with a dry one.

As soon as this bandage becomes dry, it must be re-wetted, but before replacing it, rub the beast well for at least five minutes.

This bandage is to be continued night and day and frequently changed.

Administer two clysters a day, each to consist of a quart of cold water.

Green food is best, but when this cannot be obtained, bran wetted with cold water must be substituted.

The more water drunk the better.

This treatment is to be continued until the coat looks smooth and healthy, and the appetite is regulated.

The first cold bath if carefully applied for two or three hours, will check the disease.

Two cases of cure came under notice, whilst these pages were in the press. One that of a bull of a spinal affection, and a horse with a large swelling under the belly. The bull was well rubbed all over with wet whisps, and afterwards had wet bandages, dry ones were then applied. The horse was simply bandaged, which bandages were changed when dry. He laid down the second day, which he had not done for some days before, and was well in three days.

Fits in Dogs.—Immerse the body in cold water, and let it be well rubbed until the dog recovers.

Cold water, tepid water and friction, packing sheets, the sweating process, entire baths, hip baths, foot baths, the douche, clysters and bandages, are all brought into requisition in the treatment of beasts: therefore reference should be made to the foregoing pages, in "order to understand when any one or more may be necessary." Experience proves that their effect upon man or beast is the same.

In order to give the practitioner an idea of how he might treat a horse, I subjoin the mode of treatment I adopted upon three horses belonging to a nobleman, whilst these pages were going through the press.

Monday, 19th June, 1849.—Three horses ill, two with sore throat and coughs, and one with pleurisy. Veterinary surgeon on Sunday, bled and applied mustard poultices to the latter. Monday morning, at ten o'clock, horse no better, a doubtful case. Proceeded as follows.

Took him out of the stable, drenched his whole body with many pails of cold water, then had him rubbed for several minutes with wet whisps—more water and whisps again, and finally whisped dry. Then wet sheets, wrung out, were wound round neck and body, and covered with dry ones. Before twenty minutes elapsed he was in a glow—in this state he remained for an hour and an half, when the water and friction was again repeated. When nearly rubbed dry, a sheet was doubled, wrung out in cold water, and placed round his loins, a dry one over it, and rugs put to produce a re-action. A change for the better was so evident, that the stud groom (who at first was inimical to the process being tried), declared his conviction it would cure the horse. The whole process was repeated in the evening and next morning, when the horse's appetite returned, and he was declared better. The same evening he was subjected to the packing-sheet and ablution, wore the bandage round the loins, and was cured. As the medicine, administered the day before, had acted on the bowels, I did not resort to clysters, which I otherwise should have done.

For the sore throat, one horse the first day was treated exactly as above described, but it was found unnecessary to resort to the cold ablution, previous to the packing-sheet process. A wet bandage covered with a dry one was worn round his waist and throat continually.

The third horse, having a sore throat and slight cough, only had a wet bandage with a dry one over it applied to the throat, and changed when dry.

Thus, these three horses, without a grain of physic, were cured in three or four days. The great advantages of being thus cured, are, that the cold water created an appetite, whilst drugs would have deprived the animals of it. It gave them strength, hardened the skin, and rendered them less susceptible to atmospheric influence than they were before, and produced effects the very opposite to those of drugs.

It must be obvious that this treatment had the effect of equalising the circulation.

Several years ago I treated a horse in a similar way, twice a day, for farcy, that is to say, I subjected him to the washing, rubbing, wet-sheet, and bandages, as before described: in ten days he was perfectly well. A friend of mine seeing a cow belonging to a relation of his in the last stage, had her well wetted and rubbed for an hour, put round her waist a wet blanket, and covered her up warm; in a few hours she was better. The treatment repeated a few times twice a day effected a cure.

Bandages.—The application of wet bandages, covered with dry ones round the loins, and to parts affected, after every application of the Water-cure, is most important.

These bandages must be worn day and night; during the day they should be changed whenever they become dry—it is not necessary during the night, except where there is great inflammation, the oftener they are changed the better.

Animals under treatment for fever, inflammations of any kind, should be allowed to drink as much *cold water* as they like, and eat green food.

To give a horse a hip-bath, which we call a sitz-bath, must be left to the ingenuity of the practitioner; it is of equal advantage in the treatment of horses as men, particularly in attacks of cholic inflammation, etc.

The following extract from the *Weekly Dispatch*, of July 23, 1847, confirms what is advanced in favour of water; and excites surprise that it did not lead scientific members of the medical profession to more extensive inquiry:—

"Effect of Prussic Acid on a Rabbit.—Yesterday se'nnight, Dr. Robinson, of London, delivered the third of a series of dissertations on poisons, before the Faculty, at the Maidstone Infirmary. The subject of the evening was principally corrosive sublimate—on the mode of detecting which, the learned lecturer imparted some valuable hints. At the conclusion of the dissertation, the effect of prussic acid was tried upon a rabbit. Three drops were administered from a glass (the surface of which, most probably, abstracted half of the quantity), and the animal immediately exhibited the usual symptoms—increased action of the lungs, dilatation of the pupils, and the peculiar shrill cry, which in such cases is usually indicative of immediately approaching dissolution. In order to give it a chance of recovery, however, a few drops of ammonia were administered, without apparent benefit. A constant stream of cold water was then poured upon the base of the skull and along the spine, when the animal very shortly exhibited symptoms of resuscitation. It was then wrapped in warm flannel.

In a quarter of an hour, it was sufficiently recovered to walk. Dr. Robinson had, in a former lecture, mentioned that this mode of treatment had been discovered by accident. A cat which had annoyed the apprentices of a chemist was poisoned by them with prussic acid, and thrown away for dead. By mere accident, however, it fell under a stream of water, which was pouring from a pump; the effect of which was its gradual resuscitation. Benefiting by this hint, the same means have been since successfully applied to more than one human subject who had taken prussic acid. No instance, however, had come within Dr. Robinson's knowledge where an animal had been restored after the symptoms which this rabbit exhibited; and the singularity of the case struck the faculty as being one, a knowledge of which it was desirable should be promulgated. The rabbit is now in full health and vigour.["]

www.ingramcontent.com/pod-product-compliance
Lightning Source LLC
Chambersburg PA
CBHW081156020426
42333CB00020B/2517